WHAT OTHERS ABOUT THE II CONSUMPTION PROGRAM

Author's Note: Because I am scrupulous about maintaining my clients' privacy, I am unwilling to divulge any information that might reveal their identity.

Through her program, Deena enabled me to feel in control for the first time. She taught me how to include the foods that I love the most and give up the ones around which I had difficulty controlling myself. . . . I finally set aside the constant anxiety as to whether today would be a good day or a bad day. Through the program, she enabled me to keep track of what the day would be, to plan it, to control it, and not to deprive myself of the things I loved.

I have—with continuing care and, yes, ongoing difficulty—maintained my weight between 153 and 156 pounds for the past ten years. I was 205 pounds when I first started going to Deena.

It is a daily and lifelong struggle, requiring constant awareness, and it does not get much easier. However, I do have a program, I always have a plan, and if I slip off the line, I always get back on. . . . I am sixty-eight years old and look better than I did in my forties. I owe a huge debt of gratitude to Deena. All the people I have referred to her have benefited from her program. She can tell within one month if you will be among the 85 percent of her clients who succeed. I was fortunate to be one of them. Thank you, thank you, thank you, Deena.

My sessions with Deena went beyond enlightening; they changed the way I live. I often tell people, "Deena saved my life!" . . . She gave me the opportunity to do a complete 180-degree turn in the way I was participating in my life. Perhaps the more accurate exclamation is, "Deena saved my quality of life!"

It seems the older I get, the more intensely I live in my feelings and emotions. . . .This got to the point that I was hardly able to function at any level I considered normal. It was at this point that I contacted Deena. . . . Deena's demeanor is what initially gave me hope. . . .She was direct, assertive, strong, and clear, while still maintaining a sense of warmth and nurturing. In our first session she explained to me, in concrete scientific terminology, that behaviors were only that: behaviors. They are choices. With attention, awareness, and some practice, they can be replaced. Just as behaviors were behaviors, I learned feelings were only feelings. She taught me this without taking away my right to feel all my feelings, and without dismissing or shaming what felt real to me.

While I still primarily identify with my feelings, I am grateful to have learned from Deena that this is a learned behavior, a habit, and in time it can be replaced with a new behavior. My identification with feelings is not hopeless, though it's quite exhausting in the meantime. It's been incredibly empowering to be able to recognize when I start to get carried by the undertow, to separate my actual self from my emotion … and to know that I have time to slow down and simply collect data.

This book is a gift to anyone who reads it! It provides the most effective approach to weight loss that I have ever experienced. It enabled me to lose forty pounds and gave me the tools to maintain my new weight. A vital component of its approach is the ledger in which eating is journaled, thereby producing invaluable feedback. Out of this feedback comes insight, changes in eating habits, and a path to truly successful and permanent weight loss. This is a unique book that is certainly well worth the read!

———

Dr. Deena Solomon brings her extraordinary personal and professional experience to show how she and others have battled the shame and self-defeating scripts that prevented them from achieving and maintaining a healthy weight. Powerful and moving!

—Dan Hurley, author of *Diabetes Rising*,
and contributor to the *New York Times Magazine*,
the *Washington Post*, and *The Atlantic*

Immaculate Consumption

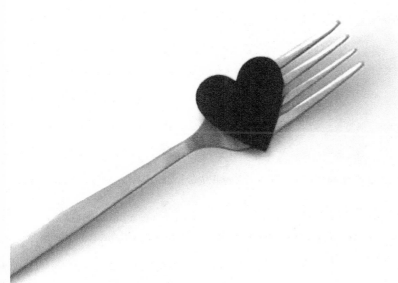

The Path to Lifelong Weight Management

Deena Solomon, PhD, MFT

IMMACULATE CONSUMPTION LIFELONG WEIGHT MANAGEMENT™
Series

Immaculate Consumption: The Path to Lifelong Weight Management

Published by Wheatmark®
2030 East Speedway Boulevard, Suite 106
Tucson, Arizona 85719 USA
www.wheatmark.com

ISBN: 978-1-62787-482-3 (paperback)
ISBN: 978-1-62787-483-0 (ebook)
LCCN: 2017930377

Cover design concept by Kathleen Mulcahy.

rev201701

To Dr. Irwin Lublin (Irv),
who provided the original inspiration for this book,
a source of academic guidance and a constant friend.

CONTENTS

Author's Note ix

Acknowledgments xi

Foreword xiii

Preface xv

Introduction 1

1 Removing Embedded Scripts 7

2 The Consultation Interview 22

3 Laying the Foundation for Self-Actualization . . . 36

4 The Downside of Linking Exercise to Weight Loss . 43

5 Cleaning out the Cobwebs 54

6 All Diets Work if You Can Stay on Them 59

7 Visible Information Is Identifiable 69

8 Data Gathering for Personalized Research 74

9 Beginning the Treatment Program 84

10 Current Behaviors Serve as Objects of Investigation . 90

11 The Initial Treatment Session 100

12 Historical Antecedents of Modern-Day Dieting . . 111

13 The Initial Treatment Session—Continued 122

14 The Third Session—The First "Uh-Oh" Moment .   . 134

15 The Fourth Week—Recovery from Regressions
and the Management of Cravings 147

16 Self-Direction 156

17 The Pink Box Revisited 165

Epilogue   171

Postscript: A Client's View of the Ledger   179

Meet Deena Solomon, PhD, MFT   181

AUTHOR'S NOTE

As I have written elsewhere in *Immaculate Consumption*, there is a single overriding factor that powers this book: how will the information provided enable you to take complete responsibility for your relationship with food?

One aspect of your responsibility is to make sure the ideas and information I am sharing with my readers are right for you. For that reason, I urge you to consult your physician and other health professionals before making use of what you find in my book.

The recommendations in this book are based on my personal experience in attaining my own weight-loss goals and maintaining my desired weight, as well as the approaches I take in helping others achieve their goals through my counseling practice. I hope my approach will be helpful to you. This is not a book of medical, nutritional, or psychological advice, and it does not take the place of a personal consultation with an appropriate healthcare professional.

Fictional names and other particulars have been used whenever I refer to an individual by first name only, with the exception of the names of my husband, Paul, and brothers, Alan and Steve. Other than those exceptions, any similarity between the fictional first names and the names of real people is strictly coincidental.

I have cited and discussed the research conducted by the National Weight Control Registry (NWCR) and others in the field of weight loss and weight maintenance. However, no affiliation with, and no endorsement by the NWCR or any other person or organization, is claimed or suggested.

I have referenced a few commercial diet programs for purposes of information and comment. Again, no claim of affiliation or endorsement is intended.

Immaculate Consumption Lifelong Weight Management™ and Path to Lifelong Weight Management™ are trademarks that I use to identify the weight-loss and weight-maintenance program described in this book as well as my other products and services.

This book is sold without warranties of any kind, and the author and publisher disclaim any liability for loss, injury, or damage based on the use of this book or its contents.

WHY I TITLED THIS BOOK *IMMACULATE CONSUMPTION*

Food, air, and water are the sacred triumvirate that allows life to happen. These elements are vital to survival. But food serves a more complex function. It also can be used to provide enormous pleasure and legitimate comfort. When used to excess, however, the evidence of this overindulgence can be striking and unhealthy and is often linked with obesity and shame. Having personally and professionally experienced years of my own anguish and that of my clients, I chose to title my book *Immaculate Consumption* because I believe it provides science-based guidance at the critical moment of consumption when taking complete responsibility for what you choose to put in your mouth is absolutely vital. For me, this moment is almost sacred and represents the cornerstone of my methodology.

ACKNOWLEDGMENTS

Every time I was about to give up, every time I hit an impasse, and every time I encountered an obstacle, Larry Greene provided invaluable guidance that inspired and spurred me on to complete this book. My husband (and country western dance partner), Paul Winnemore, provided invaluable emotional support, encouraging me when I became discouraged while providing constant love, support, and help through the difficult times. Dean Cohen's brilliant technical and creative skills made my introductory video hum. I feel fortunate having Dean in my life, confident I'll be relying on his talents in the future. Mary (Kitty) Walker has been a friend for close to four decades. During this time she has helped teach me how to make judicious decisions about taking the best possible care of myself. Kathleen Mulcahy has been a dear friend and support system throughout the journey of writing this book and has introduced me to amazing people who guaranteed that my voice was heard. One was especially important: Lisa Elia, whose professionalism, persistence, and mindfulness made me believe that I could actually become media savvy. Eleanor Winnemore, whose faith is impenetrable. A woman who, at 92, shows more energy and physical stamina than most half her age. Keeping physically and mentally fit, she's role modeled a vision of hope for the future. Finally, I want to acknowledge every single client I've worked with during all these years of clinical practice. Their trust in me through the shared trials and tribulations has provided the data and scientifically-proven methods that have been included in the following pages. Their proactive participation in the Immaculate Consumption Program has made this book possible.

FOREWORD

Immaculate Consumption: The Path to Lifelong Weight Management, is a godsend for those who have been unsuccessful with other slickly marketed commercial weight-loss programs. You know the ones that are consummately advertised on TV and show before and after photos attesting to dramatic weight loss...the ones that peddle luscious meals and hunger-busting shakes and snacks...the ones that promote their "professionally trained" consultants and/or support groups, and the ones that have famous spokespeople touting how many pounds they've lost, but not how much they're paid for their endorsements or the evidence that they may have subsequently regained the lost weight and perhaps more.

This book describes a proven scientific cognitive behavior modification program that is designed for those who have failed to lose weight or failed to keep it off. It revolves around profoundly changing your relationship with food. Unlike other programs, there are no pre-packaged foods to buy. No sign-up fees. No contracts. You simply utilize this book as a guide and apply the easy-to-learn principles that it teaches. Dr. Solomon is not using this book as a marketing tool. She is not trying to bait you to become her client, and she has no hidden agenda. She is essentially retired from private practice. She does, however, want to disseminate the insights and proprietary methods she has developed during more that thirty years of working successfully with hundreds of clients. These methods have repeatedly proven their efficacy in not only attaining weight loss but also in maintaining the weight loss. The net result is a diminishment of shame and guilt associated with having failed at another diet and a commensurate increase in self-esteem that results from having systematically achieved a heretofore elusive but cherished goal.

L. J. Greene
Educational Author

PREFACE

Deborah was everything I wanted to be. I remember that it was a balmy August morning when I went to her house. She answered the door wearing the most beautiful summer outfit I had ever seen. The buttery-colored yellow sundress fit her perfectly. Her naturally wavy hair fell gently down her back. I recall how she looked and how it awed me. Deborah had always been my idol, and I knew that as long as I did everything that she did, my joy would be assured. The year was 1953 and I was four years old.

Deborah invited me into the kitchen for a glass of freshly squeezed orange juice. Her mother gracefully poured the juice into my glass, and I put the glass up to my lips and took a long, slow sip. Never in my life had I tasted anything so wonderful. I turned around and saw Deborah running over to her father, who was sitting on a living room chair reading the morning paper. She climbed onto his lap and gave him a big hug around his neck. He chuckled while he hugged her, and he told her how much he loved her. Then he left for work.

I didn't have a buttery-colored sundress, and my family ate whole oranges that we sliced and shared among the five of us, but one thing was the same: I, too, had a dad whom I adored. Poppa had brought home a cookie jar from his hardware store when I was two years old. The jar was in the shape of a little girl with golden hair, just like me. For as long as I could remember, my dad referred to me as "My Little Cookie" whenever he pointed to the cookie jar that was on the counter near the toaster. My Little Cookie was his special pet name for me, and every time he pointed to the jar, I felt happy. I was sure that he loved me.

Having spent the morning at Deborah's house, I devised a plan for when my dad came home that evening. He would come home, and I would climb onto his lap, hug him, and tell him how much I loved him. It was so exciting for me, because I had never climbed onto his lap before. Could it be that I had just forgotten to do it? All that I knew, at that moment, was that my dad would see how much I loved him, and I would receive his love in return.

As I waited at the window that evening, I saw his blue Studebaker pull into our driveway. I rushed to hide beneath the stairway before he came into the house and waited there, excitedly, for him to sit down so that my lap sitting could take place. Poppa sat down on our comfy green chair in the living room. He took off his shoes and put on his brown leather slippers. This was the moment I had waited for, maybe for my entire life. I was thrilled about what was going to happen. Then I ran over and tried to climb onto his lap.

His reaction was quick and assertive. Dad pushed me away. He probably didn't realize how forcefully he had pushed me, but I landed on the floor. I just sat there, staring up at him. Looking down at me, he sternly said, "Deena, you're too heavy. You'll hurt my legs." That was the moment I knew, without a doubt, that my body was somehow bad. As a four-year-old, I couldn't fully comprehend what being fat meant. All I knew was that my body would have caused my beloved dad physical pain. I never tried to sit on his lap again.

This hadn't happened to Deborah. You see, she was small and petite. I was sure Deborah's dad wasn't afraid that she could possibly hurt his legs. How could she? She was so tiny.

That's when I began to compare myself to Deborah and, eventually, to everyone else. It always seemed that I was bigger than everyone around me.

My eldest brother, Alan, perceiving my emotional vulnerability, went right for the jugular. His pet name for me: "Crisco, fat in a can." The kids in the neighborhood soon became privy to Al's pet name. Oh, how they tormented me!

It was now 1957, and I was eight years old. My mother had taken me shopping for clothes in the larger children's sizes section of our local department store. I began to cry when everything I tried on was too tight. I begged my mother to help me. She took me to see our family doctor, Dr. Smoley, who handed Mom a box of crackers. I was supposed to drink three glasses of water while I ate three crackers. The rationale for this dieting procedure was that the crackers would swell in my tummy, and I would be less hungry. It didn't work. The crackers tasted like sawdust and had no effect on my appetite. Mom went out and bought some Metrecal. This was a liquid you would drink instead of a meal, and it was touted as a weight-loss miracle. We bought the chocolate flavor, which was my favorite. I ended up freezing it and eating it as a dessert after every meal. The miracle drink didn't work either; I didn't lose any weight. Life went on, and I just forgot about trying to lose weight.

It was now 1959. I was ten years old and about to enter the fifth grade. All I could think about was that Agnes, the other fat girl in my school, was going to be in my class. I was excited. You see, Agnes was heavier than I was, and I thought it obvious that a lot of attention would be diverted from me and directed to her. I also thought Agnes and I could become friends. It would be easier being friends with someone who was fat, like me.

The first day of school came on a Monday morning. I distinctly recall sitting in class waiting for Agnes to show up. I had saved a seat for her next to me. When she came through the door, the memory of Deborah came flooding back. Agnes was wearing the most beautiful off-white dress, embossed with little pink flowers and tiny green leaves. The dress was tight at the waist and had thin spaghetti straps. To my astonishment, Agnes was now thin! I mean really skinny! Agnes had one of the prettiest figures I had ever seen. The only thought that came to my mind was, "Now, I'll be the only fat kid in our class."

Agnes took the seat I had been saving for her. The moment she sat down, I begged her to tell me how she had lost all her weight. She said, "It was easy." Then she opened up her pocketbook, pulled out a small plastic pouch, and showed me some little orange pills. "Diet pills," she said. "It's so simple. I take one three times a day, and I'm never hungry." Agnes had found the weight-loss answer!

I had to get Mom to take me to the doctor for those little pills! At first, she refused. But I became a raving maniac on a weight-loss mission—a force my mother couldn't reckon with—and she eventually gave in. I was only a ten-year-old, but my doctor prescribed pure amphetamine for me. From an introverted fat kid, I became, almost overnight, an extroverted and aggressive kid who was losing over five pounds a week. I couldn't sleep at night. At the crack of dawn, I would sneak out of the house and run around the block several times—I mean, Forrest Gump-type running. I would run for hours trying to manage my excess energy.

After four weeks of taking those little pills, I went shopping for clothes with my mom again. Everything that had previously been too tight now fit perfectly. We were both elated. We couldn't stop giggling as the whole dressing room began filling up with the many outfits I was trying on. Mom bought four new dresses for me, to go with my new thin body. These were dresses we really couldn't afford, but we were both so ecstatic that money seemed to be of no concern.

At the age of ten, I had become a diet-pill junkie. During the next several years, whenever I ran out of pills, I would begin to regain the weight I had lost. I learned how to get prescriptions filled (i.e., "scored") from different doctors. I also learned to hoard my pills, guaranteeing that I could sustain my weight loss. It was relatively easy to score diet pills from doctors because it was obvious that I was a good candidate for them.

I was on and off diet pills for the next decade. Every year I would fluctuate between 130 pounds and 170 pounds, depending on whether I could get pills or not. By the mid-1960s, doctors were getting hip to diet-pill abuse. No problem. At that time, it was easy to get any kind of drug on the streets. But there were still times when I couldn't procure the pills. As a surrogate for the medication, I'd just go on one of the flavor-of-the-month diets to lose weight. I always lost weight on these diets but then quickly regained it. Eventually, I knew, I'd find someone to sell me the pills I needed to lose weight.

One day, in 1968, I realized that I had to stop abusing my body. I called my older brother Steve (the nice one), who had moved to California. I told him that I was in trouble. He never asked any questions. All he said was, "Get out to the West Coast." That was the year I stopped taking diet pills. I was nineteen years old.

Over the next few years, I ballooned up to a whopping 220 pounds, which on a five-foot-two-inch frame certainly qualified me as being morbidly obese. Because I carried this excess weight for several years, I ended up with chronic back problems, elevated blood-sugar levels, bad knees, high cholesterol, and a "weird" (as the doctor described it) heartbeat.

Every thought during every moment of every day revolved around my weight. I'd be walking past a building, and I'd see an obese person's reflection staring back at me in the window. If I wanted to get between two parked cars, I would have to turn sideways. I was chronically fatigued and perpetually angry.

I began to try every diet that came out on the market. But as soon as I stopped being vigilant about my diet, my weight loss would slow down. Eventually, the weight loss would stop. I began to reintroduce some of my old high-calorie foods. Then it would happen. I would see a cookie commercial on television. Hey, no problem. I'll just have one cookie. Yeah, right. All of a sudden, WHAM, the whole box is gone, and I'm still hungry! Slowly, the bigger clothes would move to the front of my closet again. I always kept three or four sizes in my wardrobe.

After years of yo-yo dieting, I decided to stop. Just stop trying to lose weight. Screw it. Being fat is really all I'd known my whole life. I told myself, "I guess this is just the way it's supposed to be."

In 1980, my life and my self-destructive mind-set and behaviors regarding food choices changed radically, thanks to a brilliant professor who became my mentor in graduate school. Since then, I have maintained a seventy-pound weight loss.

You're about to learn a powerful protocol that can also radically and permanently alter your life, mind-set, food choices, and overall eating behavior. The following pages will illuminate the path.

INTRODUCTION

Deidre unlocks the front door of her mother's house, opens it, and yells, "Hi, Mom. I'm here!" Sure enough, the infamous words come drifting down from upstairs. "Alice," her mother, admonishes, "Don't open the Pink Box!"

Slowly, Deidre walks through the living room toward the kitchen, and on the counter sits the Pink Box. Cautiously approaching it, like a stealth-fighter pilot vectoring in on a target, she opens it up and comes face-to-face with a seven-layer chocolate cake. Her eyes widen, and her hands begin to tremble. Even after twenty years of begging her mom not to tempt her, whenever the three-month mark arrives during one of Deidre's diets, the Pink Box appears at her mother's house. This time the three-month enticement coincidentally happens to fall on Deidra's birthday, and the box contains a birthday cake. Her confrontation with the contents of the Pink Box (whenever it appears and whatever bakery treat it contains) represents the precise moment when Deidre's dieting resolve is annihilated.

Most dieters relate to Deidre's Pink Box experience because it almost certainly parallels the trials and tribulations of their own weight-loss attempts. Seemingly insurmountable temptations present themselves and break the back of their dieting resolve.

We'll be following Deidre on her weight-loss journey. Her years of failed dieting attempts and succumbing to the lure of the iconic Pink Box exemplify how every neatly packaged diet program is irrevocably destined to fail at some point.

1

BEING SET UP TO FAIL

All diets have a common thread that preordains an eventual outcome: the inability to manage and maintain weight loss. The dieting industry fails to prepare dieters to adapt and adjust to ever-changing temptations and situations. With virtually all weight-loss programs and methods, there will come a point when you will have to face an imminent, unplanned eating event that represents nonadherence to the diet and typically starts the downward trajectory toward an unrecoverable relapse. Such seemingly impulsive yet preordained decisions trigger a chain reaction that results in psychologically destructive feelings of personal defeat. It is virtually indisputable that dieters who dare to deviate from the chiseled-in-stone dictates of their traditional diet plan are ultimately destined to compromise their own success.

The example of Deidre succumbing (over and over) to the enticement of the Pink Box underscores how virtually every diet program sets up the dieter for inevitable failure. The first deviation from the edicts of the diet might be almost unnoticeable, but rest assured, the rule violations invariably produce dire consequences. The first slip results in a shockingly private moment in the dieter's mind when he or she can no longer deny the obvious and must shamefully admit, "I've failed." Every subsequent noncompliant act compounds this initial disappointment and adds to the burden of the many letdowns the dieter has already experienced in previous dieting attempts.

Weight-loss sustainability is where virtually every diet fails miserably. This is the Achilles heel in the dieting process. Weight-loss methods that rely on willpower for getting back on track will never provide the learning skills necessary for the permanent management of your food at the moment of consumption. This can only be accomplished when going off track and being able to get back on track is strategically factored into the program.

Deidre's Pink Box moment highlights the one common denominator in essentially every dieting method—other than the one proposed in this book—namely, the lack of a method for managing the inevitable unplanned and high-calorie eating events that doom so many dieters to failure. In other programs, dieters are forced to rely on willpower and self-control tactics as the way to manage and resist temptations and non-hunger eating events.

But at some point, all the willpower in the world will not enable you to avoid an unplanned and high-calorie eating event that can derail a traditional diet. Yet through consistent application of the Immaculate Consumption Program (ICP) described in this book, you'll learn habits and develop strategies for lifelong weight management even in the face of ever-changing circumstances.

> "The real voyage of discovery consists not in seeking
> new lands but seeing with new eyes."
>
> —Marcel Proust, famous French author

TAKING A NEW PATH

Let's imagine what might happen if, one day when walking home from the local market, you discover there's been a sewer-line break that forces you to take a detour. This requires an unexpected deviation from your normal route. Okay. It's no big deal. You just need to make a minor alteration in the path you've always relied on to get home. You may be a creature of habit, but habits don't apply today. The requisite minor detour may force you slightly out of your comfort zone; it may also stir up anxiousness on the one hand and perhaps a twinge of excitement on the other. You rely on an internal map to guide you on the alternate path home. You may actually feel enlivened while taking the alternate route, because everything seems new.

Walking home becomes almost an adventure. You discover that just one little change in your daily routine heightens your senses. You never could have predicted that a simple alteration in your modus operandi would produce such a reaction. Unlocking the front door, you walk in, and all the familiar feelings of home's comfort envelop you, but this time it's different. You've experienced something unique and meaningful along the way. You're glad to be home, yet you seem to have a heightened appreciation for this safe harbor. Your journey has elicited so many new feelings that when you get home, you actually bring with you the effects of these feelings. This isn't necessarily good or bad; it's just different and refreshing. Upon further reflection, you get it. A path that always goes the same way and leads to the same place prevents you from experiencing new things from new perspectives and seeing what different options exist. The old and familiar may be comfortable, but the tried and true comfort also constitutes a rut and inhibits your ability to react flexibly to the world around you.

This little story is, of course, a metaphor. Encouraging you to deviate from the dieting path you've already followed so many times before—without success—is one aim of the weight-loss methodology you're about to learn. To be successful in attaining and maintaining your weight-loss goal, you must be willing to pursue an alternative path. But as in our metaphor, you will learn to develop an internal map to guide you on the path you will follow—an internal map uniquely suited to your personal weight-loss goal.

It may surprise you that any divergence from weight-loss goals can actually be a positive experience that provides an opportunity for an unexpected adventure that may be unusual, exciting, and daring. Unlike the process of breaking the grip of an addiction to a hard-core drug such as heroin, which requires total abstinence for success, you need food to survive. And yet, ironically, like heroin, food can also destroy your life and even kill you.

Thus, managing what you eat requires a continual decision-making process. Sometimes these decisions will be effortless. Sometimes they will require a great deal of work on your part to make reasoned and strategic choices about what food you eat. There will be stressful times, when all you might think about is stuffing your face, and by so doing, you may fixate on food and seek to indulge your cravings while retreating into a state of willful oblivion—or you might swing to the other extreme and not eat all day. You will learn that when you deviate from your goal, there is an embedded path in the Immaculate Consumption Program that will always lead you home. Predictability will be restored. You'll be confident that whenever an unpredictable or wayward situation arises (such as stress eating or pigging out at a wedding reception), you'll be able to handle it and get back on track.

Throughout the chapters that follow, the single overriding factor that powers this book is: how will the information that is provided enable you to take complete responsibility for your relationship with food? Each chapter will define the core principles that contribute to forming permanent and positive habits that facilitate losing weight and maintaining your weight loss. These principles evolved from historical and academic roots that have been extensively researched in laboratories and clinical settings for more than 150 years.

You are about to learn the clinical and practical applications of the two scientific principles that will enhance your ability not only to attain the weight-loss results you desire, but you will learn how to manage the weight you have lost throughout your life. This book will furnish you with a proven, scientifically based methodology that will guide you on the course you'll need to follow during your journey. Nonstressful, effective, rewarding, and safe travel requires that there be a competent and proactive captain at the helm, and this person is you. The decisions you make will steer and position you so you'll be able to arrive at your desired destination.

I've carefully included information for this book that will permit and encourage you to determine your own unique and personal weight-loss adventure. Yes, there are dangers and risks whenever you embark on a journey and leave the safe harbor called home. Though you may have some trepidation when you begin your trip, if you carefully plot your course and rely on two scientifically proven principles, you can procure the necessary predictability, safety, support, and comfort to sustain you during the voyage. Developing and adhering to an itinerary and applying functional travel procedures will create habits that, with practice, will help you stay on course almost automatically. Your map will become embedded and internally regulated. You just envision where you want to end up, turn toward that direction, and advance in careful increments that will ultimately bring you to your destination.

The journey you'll take with this book will help you research personal strategies that you'll always have at your disposal—strategies enabling you to adapt and adjust to every condition and situation that presents itself. You'll learn the tools that will help you develop an internal locus of control and navigate through any circumstance that might arise. By applying the tried-and-true methodology described in this book, you'll be confident that you're developing personalized and internalized food-consumption strategies that will ensure your success. The ultimate destination will be a lifelong weight-management capability.

1

♦

REMOVING EMBEDDED SCRIPTS

The last diet I was on was in 1978. The program was called Venus de Milo. After enrolling, I was assigned a diet coach who put me on a semi-starvation fast and an intensive exercise program. For eight months, I was the perfect dieter and followed a food plan of five to eight hundred calories a day. My weight dropped over sixty pounds. My blue jeans went from a size forty to a size twenty-nine.

The storefront that housed the Venus de Milo program contained some unimpressive, non-state-of-the-art gym equipment, but I didn't care. In one day, my exercise schedule increased from being virtually nonexistent to being a grueling routine of two to three hours a day, five days a week.

I was twenty-nine years old when I began the Venus de Milo program. I was caught up in a marriage that made me miserable, and I had been diagnosed with high blood pressure and high cholesterol. My height was five foot two inches, and I weighed 220 pounds. Even at this weight, I would ski at Mammoth Mountain, a resort town about five hours from Los Angeles. It would take me an hour or two to get down the mountain because I had to stop often to rest, so one run per day was all I could accomplish.

I was at one of the lowest points of my life when my friend Susan suggested we check out a local diet center. I willingly accompanied her. After we listened to the sales pitch, Susan signed up, so I just followed her lead and enrolled also. Subsequent to enrolling, we were introduced to Ellen, a fifty-year-old lady who wore exercise clothes. I immediately noticed how physically fit she was.

The very first thing Ellen did was to weigh us. The scale indicated that I weighed in at a whopping 220. In stark contrast, my friend Susan weighed 127 pounds and was five foot five inches tall. Although she didn't have any weight to lose, Susan asserted that she wanted to become healthier and more active. I suspected she was joining for my sake, but I said nothing.

After being weighed, we went over to Ellen's desk, and she pulled out a gray sheet of paper in a plastic sleeve. The gray sheet indicated that I was to drink only water, and lots of it, for the first three days. As Susan was not obese, she was given a pink sheet that detailed a much less severe diet. On the fourth day, I would be allowed one meal of spinach and eggs. This was the only food I could eat for the following two weeks. After two weeks, the only food I would be permitted to consume had to be taken exclusively from the items listed on the gray sheet of paper, and I was instructed to keep that sheet close to me at all times.

I felt dazed and confused when I left the center after that first meeting. What had I gotten myself into? After all, I had only gone along to keep my friend company; I hadn't given any serious thought to the implications. My need to be thin seemed to have vanished the day I got married. I was with a man who didn't seem to care what I looked like, so why should I? Yet I had just signed up for a program that I really couldn't afford in the first place.

My head was screaming, "Go back in and tear up the contract!" The only thing stopping me was the feeling that I couldn't disappoint my friend or the trim gym-clothes-wearing lady. If I tore up the contract, they wouldn't like me anymore. I had learned at an early age that being fat meant you had to be extra nice to people, or they wouldn't want to be friends with you. I was left with no choice.

Almost immediately, I became addicted to losing weight. The scale was going down really fast, and I lost forty pounds very quickly. I told Ellen that going to the bathroom was becoming increasingly difficult. It was comforting to hear that this was normal when losing weight, and she suggested I take some laxatives to solve my problem. This advice was a godsend that helped alleviate my constipation immediately, but I eventually found it such a trial to limit my daily food intake to the prescribed five hundred calories that whenever I exceeded the limit and ate extra food, I'd just get rid of the caloric evidence of my cheating by taking extra laxatives. After a while, my high calorie consumption days were becoming more and more frequent, and keeping my weight under control was requiring a great deal of effort, willpower, and, of course, laxatives.

Since I had been overweight and had felt unattractive most of my life, dating and romance were issues I never even seriously thought about. In 1971, a man asked me for my hand in marriage. I married my first husband simply because he asked. It was a difficult marriage from the start, but he had accepted me and my obesity, which was the number one priority for me. In 1978, I began to lose weight via the Venus de Milo program. With every pound I lost, my husband seemed to get angrier and angrier. Looking back now, I realize that my obesity had made him confident that other men would stay away. Also, my obesity complemented his entrenched lifestyle of eating ice cream, pizza, and candy every night while watching television.

We hadn't lived as man and wife for years, and after I lost a significant amount of weight, I made the first of many decisions that would ultimately end in our divorce. I asked him to move to the downstairs bedroom. He did so willingly and without a fight. My weight was down in the 150-pound range, and my energy level had skyrocketed. Since it was becoming impossible to come home to a man who was so angry at me all the time, I decided to do one of the things I loved the most: go dancing.

Technically I was still married, but in actuality, men terrified me. I just wanted to dance. I had no interest in going to a bar to drink and meet men, and in the late 1970s, bars were one of the only places to dance. Until that point in my life, all I knew about love and romance was what I'd learned from movies, television, or books. This situation was just fine with me, since guys had always made fun of me because of my weight, but I still really wanted to get out and dance.

Fortuitously, the 1980 movie *Urban Cowboy* had just come out, and it created a boom for pop-country music. Many clubs that were once disco bars were now offering country-western dancing. Line dancing was the rage and perfect for what I was looking for. With line dancing, you don't have to rely on being asked to dance; you just join in with the crowd.

There was a dance club, formerly a disco, close to where I lived. It was a takeoff on Gilley's Dance Hall in Pasadena, Texas, a spot made popular by the aforementioned movie. This club near me, in Marina Del Rey, offered country-western dancing seven days a week, and just like Gilley's, it had a mechanical bull. Not wanting to go on my very first dance-club excursion alone, I asked my older brother Steve to go with me. He always took good care of me, and he was the person with whom I felt the safest. I stood at the edge of the dance floor and watched the crowd of "cowboys" and "cowgirls" dancing the two-step, a dance made popular by the movie. The song everyone was dancing to was "Lookin' for Love" by Johnny Lee.

In retrospect, the song seems prescient. Just as I was thinking that I had never looked for love before (and obviously had never found it), this cowboy suddenly grabbed my hand and dragged me out onto the dance floor. He asked, "Do you two-step?" Terrified, I just said, "No." Looking straight into my eyes, he said, "You're about to learn the most romantic dance ever invented." I found myself on the dance floor looking into the face of a Robert Redford lookalike. As soon as I began to breathe again (after managing my shock), I realized I was totally smitten by my two-stepping cowboy. It was pure, unadulterated love.

Since I wasn't familiar or comfortable with feelings of sexual tension and attraction, it was impossible for me to admit what had really transpired: I had just fallen head over heels in lust for the first time in my life. Reluctantly, I left the club a few hours later at my brother's insistence, but knowing that I'd be returning tomorrow made leaving a little easier.

Movies had provided me with a fantasy life resplendent with vicarious love, romance, and adventure. In my attempts to understand feelings that I'd never personally experienced, I relied on movie scenes, such as when Clark Gable grabbed and kissed a seemingly unwilling Vivian Leigh in *Gone with the Wind*, or when Richard Burton demanded Elizabeth Taylor submit to him in *Taming of the Shrew*. The scripts were with me constantly, but the difference now was that the characters were real, and it wasn't a fantasy. Reflecting on the moment when my cowboy pulled me onto the dance floor caused many sleepless nights during the next weeks. Oh, the delicious pain of love.

I wanted to make sure I'd have a replay with my cowboy, so when I got home that night, I took my fifteen-year-old Frye boots out of the closet and dusted them off. I went shopping the next day and found a Western-type white-eyelet button-down blouse with tiny pearls sewn into it. The collar had a little black cord bowtie. I would tuck this blouse into the twenty-nine-inch waist of my Levi 501 blue jeans. This outfit would guarantee my acceptance into the Cowgirls Club in Marina Del Rey, California.

Sure enough, my fantasy was realized the next evening when my cowboy was ready and willing to continue my two-step lessons. I quickly became one of the best dancers in the club. Whether line- or couples dancing, I was always on the dance floor. In a little over a week, my obsession with country-western dancing was in full swing. Like a moth drawn to flame or a bee drawn to honey—or, for that matter, a junkie drawn to heroin—my addiction to the urban country movement defined most of my social life for the next few years. The vision of riding off into the sunset with my Marina Del Rey cowboy kept me romantically entertained for months.

Looking back, it's easy for me to appreciate how cults grab hold of people who are looking for companionship and a community to identify with. I was among a group of like-minded people who shared a passion for and dedication to the country-western movement.

The club in Marina Del Rey had names for all the dances, and when a song played, we all knew the specific dance for that tune. There were dress codes for different days of the week. Wednesday was Hawaii night, and everyone in our group showed up wearing some kind of Polynesian shirt. On Wednesdays, if someone showed up *not* wearing a Polynesian shirt, our group knew immediately that the person didn't belong. The Hawaiian shirt I had bought several years earlier served me in good stead. Wearing it was another sign that I belonged to the core group.

Unlike the past, when I'd stick out like a sore thumb wherever I went because of my weight, now whenever I came into the club, someone always had a seat waiting for me. It took some time for me to walk into the club without expecting to hear, "Oink, oink, here's the fat girl." Finally, I was seen as a well-dressed woman, a dancer, an attractive girl, a student—or I was described in other typically superficial, yet normal, everyday bar lingo. I walked in one Friday night and had an overwhelming feeling of gratitude when I realized I was a regular human being who fit in perfectly. I was no longer stigmatized because of my weight.

When I went to the gym one day, I got on the scale, and it read 139 pounds! For the first time since the age of twelve, I was out of the 140s. I had seen a picture of a Laura Ashley dress in a magazine several weeks earlier, and this was the day I'd finally buy that dress. I had never heard of this designer before, but to me, the dress looked like it came straight out of the Old West. I knew immediately it was my dress, and to allay my impatience, I had had to assure myself it would be just a matter of time before I could afford it. For the last few years, I had been living exclusively on student loans, but I had recently accepted my brother's invitation to waitress at his new restaurant, and this enabled me to begin treating myself to a few extra luxuries. Even though it would be a hardship, I had managed to save some money, and this was the day I planned to shell out $189 for that dress.

The store was in Beverly Hills. When I showed the picture of the dress to the saleswoman, she brought me over to where it was hanging and took down a size ten.

"Oh no," I said, "that's too small. It will never fit."

"Trust me," she replied. "I know sizes." Then, "Wait," she said, handing me a white slip. "A petticoat is a must for wearing under that dress."

I asked if petticoats were worn in the Old West.

She smiled and said, "Petticoats, or waist slips as they were first called, were introduced in 1585 in England."

Then I asked if this style of dress was from the Old West.

"No, dear," she gently replied with a smile, "Laura Ashley is a Welsh fashion designer. This style of clothing is based on rural communities from the English countryside in the eighteen hundreds."

I easily zipped up the dress in the changing room and slipped on the petticoat under it. White eye-lit ruffles hung about a half-inch below the dress.

When I came out, the well-groomed saleslady said, "This dress was designed with you in mind."

My first thought (apparently betrayed by my facial expression) was, "Sure, you just want a sale."

She looked me in the eyes and said, "My dear, you look like an innocent country maiden in that dress. In the seven years I've worked here, never has anyone looked better in it."

"Thank you," I told her. I said I'd take the dress but couldn't afford the petticoat.

She insisted that she couldn't possibly let me wear that dress without the petticoat, adding, "Let the waist slip be a gift on me, but there's one condition. When that person you're wearing it for asks for your hand in marriage, send me an invitation."

"It's a deal," I replied.

When I walked into the club that Friday evening, all eyes turned in my direction.

"Uh oh," I thought, "I must look ridiculous." Then, my Robert Redford came over and held out his hand to dance to what the band was playing, "The Cowboy Waltz."

While we moved around the dance floor, he asked if I'd like to go for a cup of coffee Sunday night after dancing. There was a twenty-four-hour diner next to the club, but because Monday was a workday, Sunday night at the club was usually an early evening for most of us. Since speaking was out of the question, I just nodded. My cowboy smiled.

"Cloud nine," the commonly heard expression, was thought to originate from the classification of fluffy cumulonimbus clouds that most people consider delicate and attractive. Another explanation derives from Buddhism, in which the cloud nine is one stage of progression toward enlightenment for the bodhisattva, one destined to become a Buddha.

My own cloud nine was certainly not of this world. Falling asleep that night, all I could think about was what I'd wear for my wedding. I quickly decided on a Laura Ashley dress, of course. The warm feeling in my tummy soon emanated throughout my body. Sleep came easily, and the delicious dreams of love soothed me all night long. Then, in the morning, the worst possible thing happened.

THE DAY THE EARTH STOOD STILL

Saturday was my usual weigh-in day at Venus de Milo, and afterward, I'd begin my three-hour routine on the machines. I got dressed for my Saturday weigh-in and workout, then drove to the facility. The door refused to open. I began to yank on it, hard. Then I saw it: a tiny, handwritten note stating, "Closed due to bankruptcy."

My mouth didn't shut for at least two minutes. "Wait," I thought in a moment of absolute panic, "who's going to weigh me in? Who's going to cheer me on while I'm sweating on the machines? Where the hell are my before and after pictures?"

I had never felt more alone in my life. At that instant, my only option was to sit down on the curb. I began to cry, then sob. My whole body shook. Soon, I couldn't breathe. I had never had an anxiety attack before, and my first one was a doozy.

Everyone at Venus de Milo had been so nice to me. I really felt they liked me. Each person there had a specialized job that helped me stay on track with my diet as they told me what to eat and what exercise routine to do each time I arrived. My faith in Venus de Milo and reliance on this center had been complete and unquestioning. Who could I possibly rely on now to tell me what to do?

My head hung down as I walked over to my car. Shocked, confused, and completely lost, I sat in the car and stared at the empty storefront. Then, feelings of pure terror began to emerge. Without any diet plan that day, I began to realize how ravenous I was.

As the shock wore off, my warrior side took over. My gray sheet hadn't been necessary during the last several months, and I had relegated it to a kitchen drawer. After retrieving it from the drawer, I taped it securely to the front of the refrigerator at eye level.

"I can do this," I told myself with assurance. I realized that resisting the food at my brother's restaurant would be difficult, but I felt I could do it. I made a deal with myself right then and there that whenever I walked into the restaurant, I'd just rely on "old faithful," spinach and eggs—the food that had gotten me to where I started on my weight-loss journey. I thought, "This is going to work!" And it did work, for one whole day.

The following morning, I needed to show up early to get ready for the breakfast crowd when the doors of Steve's restaurant opened at 7:00 a.m. Upon opening the door, I was immediately attacked by the aroma of frying bacon. Bacon! It was certainly not on my gray sheet. Perhaps you've seen the television commercial where a golden retriever is running from room to room yelling, "Bacon! Bacon! Bacon!" In my mind, I was running alongside him, fearful that I'd actually run over the dog to reach the treat first.

On my coffee date with my cowboy that evening, as I looked into his dreamy eyes, my only thought was, "I wish I hadn't binged this morning on those fifteen pieces of bacon."

I was soon heaping on the calories. Alone, with no one to report to, my food consumption was now completely unmanageable. Fortunately, laxatives were easily available. What started as a once- or twice-a-week practice—using laxatives to get rid of caloric evidence—quickly became a daily ritual.

Realizing I needed help, I began going to meetings for people who had problems with food. The groups were leaderless, and the people who attended were terrific. Everyone would nod in agreement and acknowledge each other's eating trials and tribulations. The belief was that by going public with personal food challenges and tragedies, shame would be dispelled and self-loathing absolved.

One night, a girl stood up and said she had to confess something that she had never told anyone. Standing there with tears running down her face, she said, "When I eat a lot of food, I get rid of it by throwing up." I just sat there thinking, "What a much better solution; it's the perfect alternative to taking laxatives." Finally, I could give my tush a much-deserved rest.

Despite all the ways I offset my overeating, my weight slowly rose from 139 pounds, my lowest, to 149 pounds. My twenty-nine-inch waist grew to thirty and then thirty-one. I was still dancing every night, but it became apparent the day would soon come when the real Deena—the fat girl—would ultimately reappear.

My Laura Ashley dress didn't fit anymore, and I had to put it in the back of the closet. I couldn't even look at it. My life was in constant turmoil, and after a few snubs to my cowboy, he kept his distance. I had to detach myself in case a quick exit strategy was needed.

I thought the old Deena had been massacred. The new Deena's life had nothing in common with my old life as an obese person, but it was becoming obvious that my old self was getting ready to emerge once again. My last thought at night and my first thought in the morning was that I couldn't go back to my old life. Returning to the two-hundreds meant giving up everything in my current lifestyle and returning to the life of being "nonhuman." Now that I'd tasted life as a nonobese person, the thought of this happening to me once again was intolerable.

UNPACKING THE MIND OF A DIETER

Remember Susan, the friend and fellow graduate student who joined the Venus de Milo program as a subterfuge to get me to join also? She saw the depressed state I was in. After our last class one day, she told me about a professor at our university who was a psychologist and supervised a weight-loss program. That's all I needed to hear.

It was September 1980. I remember the precise time: 2:49 p.m. By 3:00 p.m., I was knocking on Dr. Irwin Lublin's office door. Actually, I wasn't just knocking. It was more like I was banging on the door with two fists and screaming "Let me in!" This is just a bit of an exaggeration, but not much. A slim man, about five foot eight inches tall, with a mustache and glasses, opened the door.

Without further ado, I said, "I'm in trouble with food, and I heard you can help."

He calmly replied, "Come in."

I entered Dr. Lublin's office and sat down. Every bit of space was taken up with paraphernalia indicating that he was a highly educated person. I realized, of course, that he was an academic and a full-time tenured professor whose therapeutic specialty was helping people with weight loss. But the only thing I really knew about this man was that he was a psychologist who had developed a weight-loss method he called Life-Long Weight Reduction. I assumed that, in addition to his teaching responsibilities, he also maintained a private practice.

Then it hit me. Sitting in this office at this time with this highly trained specialist was exactly where I was supposed to be. I intuitively sensed that Dr. Lublin could provide the help I desperately needed at this juncture in my life. That's when I panicked. Knowing full well what a psychologist charges for private therapy, I realized that I couldn't possibly afford to hire him.

When he asked me why I was there, my first and only thought was to convince him not only to take me on as his patient but also to take me on for no fee. Dr. Lublin was about to hear the spontaneous and unfiltered disclosures of someone whom (I hoped) he would find to be the most authentic and honest patient he could ever conceivably treat.

Fortunately, I could draw upon the university course I was taking at the time; it dealt with free-association, the core concept of psychoanalysis. This concept is considered a journey of co-discovery in which neither the therapist nor the patient is in control of where conversations will lead. The therapeutic procedure is predicated on the belief that by relating whatever comes into your mind and not censoring your thoughts or feelings, positive psychological growth and behavioral change will result. I was convinced that my whole future depended on my ability to show Dr. Lublin how motivated I was to make changes. Demonstrating my free-association skills would surely clinch the deal.

From my own graduate-school background and clinical experiences as an intern counseling undergraduate students, I had learned that people who are motivated to make changes are worth their weight in gold to a therapist, because they're exciting to treat. This was my chance to show Dr. Lublin how much satisfaction he would derive from working with me. Surely my obvious desperation and gratitude would be sufficient payment for him.

So, when Dr. Lublin asked, "Why are you here?" I responded the only way I knew—by free-association disclosure of all the reasons I was in his office. During the next three hours, I interspersed talking with weeping and then more talking.

I began to cry when I described my reaction to the bankrupt sign posted on the front door of the Venus de Milo facility. He just sat there, calmly looking at me. He didn't even offer me a tissue. We sat in his little office, and he listened as I told him that at four years old my dad pushed me to the floor when I tried to sit on his lap and said, "Deena, you're too heavy. You'll hurt my legs." There was still no response from Dr. Lublin.

I quickly—but, as I later discovered, erroneously—surmised that Dr. Lublin was from the Freudian school of psychology, which employed the tabula rasa or "blank slate" protocol based on Freud's insistence that a lack of demonstrable emotional involvement on the part of the analyst was imperative. This encouraged the patient's unconscious to be projected onto the passive therapist and thereby brought into the open.

Dr. Lublin was a very skilled listener. By not responding, he was obviously making sure that his thoughts or feelings would not invade the session and thereby affect his patient's ability to bring out unconscious thoughts during the free-association process. His passive silence, however, posed no obstacle for me. I began filling up the room in the only way I knew how—by talking nonstop, with time-outs for weeping.

I recounted how I ran out of my kindergarten class never to return, thanks to an abusive teacher. I related that, even to this day, the abusive teacher had left me with academic scars and classroom phobias that caused weeks of sleeplessness before the start of every school year. I talked about the person who taught me that I was fat, my verbally abusive eldest brother, Alan. His moniker for me, "Crisco, fat in a can," still haunts me to this day. Finally, Alan's verbal abuse was the reason that, at the age of ten, I begged my mom to get me the same diet pills the other heavy girl in school had taken to get thin—diet pills that turned out to be amphetamines. I disclosed to Dr. Lublin that, when I got older and couldn't get the pills from a doctor, I went to the street to score them and was subsequently introduced to cocaine. I told Dr. Lublin that a drug addiction caused me to leave school at sixteen, and I admitted the shameful fact that "I'm actually a high school dropout."

Throughout all my ranting and raving, he just sat there without even a head nod for the entire three hours. Wow, I thought, Sigmund Freud would be very proud of Dr. Lublin's consummate blank-slate stare!

Finally, I was all talked out. My soliloquy was over, and we both sat in silence looking at each other. Then he uttered the words that would change my life forever. He simply said, "Deena, you're in a master's program at California State University, Los Angeles. You're not a high school dropout anymore."

"Huh?" I thought incredulously as I struggled to wrap my mind around his simple statement.

The only way to relate what happened to me is to describe a scene from the 1984 movie *The Karate Kid*. There's a moment in the movie when the teenage protagonist, Daniel, gets pissed off after having had enough of being Mr. Miyagi's slave during the unorthodox karate training regimen: washing and waxing his instructor's cars, sanding the outside deck, and painting Mr. Miyagi's whole house. Every task has to be performed in a very specific way. Hand, wrist, and arm movements have to be done exactly the way Mr. Miyagi shows him.

After Daniel's temper tantrum about waxing the car, Mr. Miyagi yells,

"Show me: wax on, wax off!" Then, "sand floors," and finally, "paint the fence." Daniel rolls his eyes and reluctantly obeys, precisely recreating the movements that his mentor had demonstrated and that Daniel had been performing during the grueling work. Then Mr. Miyagi abruptly attacks Daniel, making the aggressive sounds and moves of someone skilled in martial arts. Daniel effortlessly averts his attacker. Then it happens—the moment when Daniel suddenly realizes that the entire time he had spent waxing, sanding, and painting, he had actually been learning karate. He had been oblivious to the fact that his mentor was teaching him the foundational movements of unarmed combat that comprise the cornerstone of the ancient martial art, which originated in Okinawa during the fourteenth century.

With obvious newfound reverence and belated insight, Daniel, while keeping eye contact at all times, reverently bows. He has found his teacher.

The very first time I met with Dr. Lublin, feelings of confusion, agitation, and turmoil had been creating chaos and havoc in my life. How do you talk down someone who is in such a state of chaos? He knew, and I now know: you can't. He wasn't creating an atmosphere based on the theory of a tabula rasa, nor was he attempting to help my unconscious become conscious by not responding. He actually didn't give a damn about any of that. He wasn't interested in any feelings or emotions I brought into the room that day, conscious or not. I was about to be apprised of the fact that Dr. Lublin wasn't a traditional *talk* therapist. He was from the opposite end of the continuum.

Dr. Lublin was a *behaviorist*, and as such, feelings and emotions were not something he paid attention to. I came into his office bringing with me an emotional forest fire raging out of control. The priority for a highly skilled behaviorist—and Dr. Lublin was one—is to put out the flames. Since the match that started the flames will always be there, talk therapists devote their energies to figuring out with their patients the underlying sources of the fire. As a behaviorist, Dr. Lublin's job was to extinguish one of the flames by dowsing it with an indisputable fact—namely, that my identity was no longer defined by dropping out of high school at the age of sixteen.

I had been in this psychologist's office for over three hours, crying and sobbing. In one fell swoop, Dr. Lublin eradicated a belief I had held since

1965—that my persona was somehow indelibly flawed. With the intake of a breath, I could finally allow myself to be awed by my subsequent academic accomplishments. I was able to consciously remind myself that, in 1967, as a night student at Flushing High School in New York City, I had belatedly earned my high school diploma. It was something I had disregarded for many years.

THE NUTS AND BOLTS OF BUILDING A FUNCTIONAL SYSTEM

After decades of feeling like an academic failure, all the feelings of self-loathing and diminished self-esteem regarding my school performance suddenly disappeared. The chaotic feelings I brought into Dr. Lublin's office that day had been replaced by one undeniable fact: "I am not a dropout today." Yes, Dr. Lublin was listening, and I discovered that my initial assumption was wrong. He was not creating a Freudian tabula rasa. Rather, as a behaviorist, he was deliberately extinguishing a chaotic and problematic thought and replacing it with an indisputable, and thus scientific, fact. I had experienced firsthand how to bring science into the clinical setting.

Before I left his office, Dr. Lublin explained that eating behaviors are embedded habits. Through repetition, I had learned my food habits. Rather than relying on the medical model of disease—where overeating is defined as an illness that must be cured—Dr. Lublin made it clear that I needed to relearn certain habits that were counterproductive to attaining my goals, which were losing weight and keeping it off.

Some background is in order. In 1963, Dr. Lublin began researching and developing the foundational system from which I subsequently derived the Immaculate Consumption Program. Dr. Lublin's Life-Long Weight Reduction treatment program evolved from his own research and from learning principles regarding habit formation that had been researched for more than 150 years, beginning with the famous Russian scientist Pavlov, who was awarded the Nobel Prize in 1904 for his meticulous empirical laboratory studies about the effects of stimuli on animal behavior. The data produced by this research revealed unequivocally that habits are learned and become embedded over time.

When I left Dr. Lublin's office, I felt immense relief that stood in stark contrast to the paralyzing fear and powerlessness I had experienced that disastrous day when I was stranded on the sidewalk in front of the locked Venus de Milo facility. Rather than feeling dazed, confused, and bereft, I had no doubt whatsoever that this man was going to help me learn, apply, and attain new habits to change my past and current eating behaviors and prepare me for a future of having more control over my food. Though I had just met him, my intuitive trust in Dr. Lublin was absolute. I now had a foretaste of how real science could be applied clinically to produce profoundly positive behavioral consequences.

As was the case with Daniel, I had found my teacher and an effective and proven method for attaining my goals. Hopefully, by committing to and engaging in the easy-to-learn and easy-to-apply procedures described in this book, you will find yours too. All the work you'll be doing with this book to alter your counterproductive eating habits is based upon two key scientific principles that regulate how learning occurs. The chapters that follow will introduce you to these two key principles and will provide you with a verified, systematic methodology for applying them in your own unique weight-loss program.

2

♦

THE CONSULTATION INTERVIEW

The majority of clients I meet for the first time bring with them the residue of all the trials and tribulations of their past dieting attempts. Most often, fear, negative expectations, discouragement, and despair overshadow any hope they might have of ever losing weight and keeping it off.

The dieting industry creates advertising programs that take advantage of desperate people who are trying to lose weight. The marketing is designed to sell a quick-fix product or service, rather than a holistic method people can use to permanently change their eating behaviors and thereby control and manage their weight over the long term.

To date, every method that promises weight-loss success has repeatedly exploited consumers because of the method's deliberately and strategically designed symbiotic structure. Consumers have to remain in the program and/or continue to buy the pills or the packaged food products to maintain any weight loss they achieve using the dieting program to which they subscribe. In effect, these programs rely on methodologies that are ultimately destined to fail because they don't permanently alter the consumer's entrenched, maladaptive eating choices and behaviors.

The primary goal of the initial consultation interview I employ is to counter the client's erroneous preconception that dieting is the only way to lose weight. For those with an extensive dieting history, it will be impossible during this first meeting to neutralize completely the feelings of shame brought about by past dieting failures. This neutralization process must be attained incrementally through the systematic course of the Immaculate Consumption Program (ICP).

When given the opportunity to meet clients face-to-face, I can usually begin to deconstruct the defense mechanisms of even the most forlorn and defeated clients and assist them in reorienting their embedded belief systems. This transformation will inexorably lead them to more productive eating choices and behaviors. A concomitant goal of the consultation interview is to furnish disheartened dieters with the opportunity to make one final proven and scientifically based venture to permanently lose weight.

I encourage their willingness to make this last effort by deliberately not charging a fee for the initial consultation. This is not a sales ploy. Rather, it is an opportunity for me to lay on the table my program, my data, and my credentials and to allow for a frank discussion of the merits and methodology of the ICP, with no strings attached. The potential client is free to reject the program, and I am also free to reject the potential client as being unsuitable.

The no-fee consultation interview simply makes it more likely that motivated, albeit tentative, potential clients will reach out. The message is: if you are willing to make an appointment, want my help, and are willing to accept my guidance, I'm here for you. The no-fee visit creates a "nothing to lose" attitude for disillusioned dieters, prompting them to make a last-ditch effort at turning their lives around before succumbing to what they may erroneously perceive as their preordained fate, namely this: that for them, being overweight is seemingly chiseled in stone or, as I used to believe, "just the way it's supposed to be."

My typical referrals come from people I've treated or from health professionals familiar with my program. Receiving an endorsement of the ICP's proven, science-based methods from a trusted source is frequently the catalyst that encourages demoralized potential clients to take the plunge. They usually want to start the program immediately, and they don't hesitate to inform me of their personal sense of urgency.

When talking with a client on the phone and trying to set up an appointment for the consultation, I often hear, "Dr. Solomon, I've met and spoken to many people about the work you do. Most of them have lost weight and kept it off for years. I know your program works, and I'm eager to begin. I'm aware of your waiting list, and I don't need to be talked into anything. I don't require the free session, so please let's just schedule our first real appointment so I can start right away."

First-time callers can't possibly grasp that they're actually about to become a researcher who will be learning how to conduct a personalized experiment in weight loss and long-term weight management. As a would-be researcher, it's imperative that the client be prepared to follow guidelines for what defines a valid scientific experiment—including reproducible results and the ability to make accurate, causal predictions. A research study is considered valid only if the outcome data unequivocally contributes to the attainment of effective and permanent changes being sought.

My response to clients who want to circumvent my standard initial intake procedure is to tell them: "Motivation has been proven the strongest indicator of future success. So while I applaud your enthusiasm, eliminating the consultation session is impossible, since this is when the inner workings of the program will be discussed. During this session, the behavior-based methodologies of the Immaculate Consumption Program are presented and integrated with the underlying scientific principles. So, skipping the consultation interview is absolutely out of the question."

THE DYNAMICS OF THE CONSULTATION INTERVIEW

As I have a home office, I've always refused to advertise my professional services. Therefore, I'm unknown to the average dieter. This relative obscurity is in stark contrast to the typical commercial weight-loss programs that are supported by multimillion-dollar advertising campaigns with marketing objectives focused on making the program visible and easily accessible. My clients usually come from a very select referral population: healthcare professionals and current or former clients. Because of my anonymity, it takes a great deal of initiative to get to see me, and potential clients have to exert themselves to procure my business card or phone number. Then, they must be ready to act on the information and make the call for an appointment, despite having to handle any emotional baggage they may be carrying with them about their weight and previous dieting attempts.

The vast majority of those seeking to lose weight have experienced repeated failures, and they carry a pervasive sense of emotional and spiritual defeat. These people have given up, because they've been ensnared and victimized by a six-hundred-billion-dollar-a-year dieting industry that promises weight loss, but over the long term has more than a 95 percent failure rate for weight-loss sustainability.

Rather than attribute their lack of success to the intrinsic limitations of the commercialized and aggressively marketed diet programs or over-the-counter "magical" appetite-suppressing or calorie-burning diet pills they've been seduced into buying, the clients referred to me typically blame themselves and their own inadequacies for their repeated failures. They've simply been disappointed and disillusioned too many times by flawed dieting schemes and the famous media stars hired to promote the slick programs.

The discouraged people I work with have endured so much yo-yo dieting that they've become convinced no weight-loss method will work for them. They've become so scarred by the negative outcomes they've repeatedly experienced that they either actively or passively resist making more sustained efforts. The population I work with has greater feelings of desperation and hopelessness than the average dieter.

A few prospective clients have actual phobias about the possibility of another disappointment and refused to contact me even after talking with satisfied friends or personally interacting with ICP graduates who have successfully attained and maintained their weight-loss goal for years.

Other prospective clients are just not good candidates for what I offer: those who lack the ability to take personal responsibility for their behaviors. On the surface, their weight-loss rationale appears plausible: "Of course I want to lose weight and learn how to keep it off." They may profess that they want to attain their goal weight, but it's questionable whether they're willing to do what it takes to get there. For whatever reasons, these people are not ready to learn and implement the self-management strategies taught in the ICP. My heart breaks for them, but I am powerless to help them until they are willing and ready to fully engage in the program.

This brings us to the second primary goal of the consultation interview: to determine the candidate's current capability to commit to the ICP protocol. The profile of the research subject (i.e., the client) is the fundamental issue in determining whether the results of the experiment will be reproducible. Outcome studies that are reproducible (i.e., methodologies that can be replicated and produce consistent results) are the only ones that allow the researcher to make accurate causal connections in the process of identifying goals and learning how to attain them. It's my responsibility to determine from the onset if potential research subjects—clients—are suitable candidates for the ICP methodology I offer.

Linda is an example of someone who would probably not prove to be a good candidate for the ICP. She contacted me because of a colleague's weight-loss success and endorsement of the program. When I spoke with her on the phone, she seemed excited to learn about the program, and she wanted to schedule an appointment "as soon as possible." We scheduled the consultation interview for the following week. When I gave her directions to my office, her response was, "Oh, that's too far. Isn't there anyone closer who does what you do?" I told her, "No, I'm the only one who does what I do." Still, she complained about the distance. The message she delivered was that the thirty-minute drive would be a hardship.

This type of response is not uncommon. It usually derives from negative associations with previous unsuccessful diet regimes, along with cumulative feelings of stress and from anticipation of ultimate and unavoidable disillusionment. One of the objectives of the consultation interview is to sort through an array of emotional baggage that potential candidates carry with them. Linda's reaction suggested that she was so psychologically and emotionally exhausted by her past dieting failures that she was unwilling to put herself through any excess inconvenience (in her case a thirty-minute drive), because she held little or no hope of success. That she was willing, however tentatively, to make the call attests to the fact that the embers of hope can rarely be completely extinguished in the human spirit.

During the phone call, I needed to decipher what Linda's motivation was for the "driving hardship" excuse. Was there a genuine feeling of futility that made her unwilling to subject herself to the minor inconvenience of the drive to my office? Or was her ambivalence symptomatic of something more deeply rooted that was stopping her from benefitting from the methodology I was offering? What was her real message? The underlying emotional components of Linda's ambivalence defined the essential personality qualities that made her who she was at that moment in her life.

Her answer to the following question provided a clue about how Linda would react to current and future events. I asked her (and you must ask yourself): "On a scale from zero (being completely unimportant) to ten (being the most important thing in your life), what number would you assign for getting down to your goal weight and staying there the rest of your life?" The answer to the question indicates when and if someone is truly ready to commit to doing what's required in the ICP so they can ultimately take complete responsibility for their eating decisions and behaviors.

For whatever reason, Linda replied, "Seven." I was gentle, yet insistent, when I told her, "When it gets to a ten, give me a call." An answer less than ten clearly suggests that someone is externally—rather than internally—motivated and therefore less likely to succeed in the program.

Her colleague's success had been the prime motivation for Linda to call me, but she was simply going through the motions. Linda's fiery motivation was quickly doused by her justification about how inconvenient the drive would be. My clinical instincts told me that she was probably not capable of taking responsibility to do what was necessary to develop new eating habits. The distance factor was an example of an external excuse to get herself off the hook. She would be inclined to use it to rationalize her failure to act.

Other prospective clients who have proven to be unsuitable candidates for the ICP are those who tell me during the initial call something like: "My doctor told me that if I don't lose fifty pounds, I'm going to die!" A big red flag immediately goes up and flaps in the wind. I have found that these referrals are typically the least compliant, arrive late and/or cancel appointments, and are generally the quickest to drop out of the program. Why? First, they're following and complying with their highly respected doctor's orders, which represents an external motivation. Second, those who might potentially die of their obesity-related medical conditions are often incapable of recognizing and/or unwilling to recognize the damage their continual food overconsumption is doing to their physical health, which represents a lack of internal motivation to rectify the situation.

In contrast, the most successful clients are those with internal motivations for losing weight. They might say, "I want to lose weight because of what I see when I look into a mirror," or "I want to buy a knockout wardrobe." Tangible goals are more likely to be attained than intangible ones, and internal motivations produce greater long-term success than external ones.

Then there are those who are good candidates for the ICP, but for whatever reason, it's just not the right time to start. Several years ago, a man was referred to me who said his wife told him that lovemaking was out of the question until he lost weight and became attractive again. Marvin was very motivated to feel better about himself (internal motivator), but he declared that he was also motivated to please his wife (external motivator). His motivation to lose weight was a mixture of internal and external motivations, which was a yellow flag for me.

Marvin began the program and was successfully working toward his weight-loss goal, but his wife continually reproached him when he was about to eat. She would scream, "Is that on your diet?" After three weeks, he came in and admitted that he was primarily trying to lose weight to please his wife and not himself. Because of her perpetual abuse, he began to resent the program's protocol. I tried to return his first month's check, to which he replied, "Dr. Solomon, after seeing my friend keep off weight for years, combined with my short involvement, it's obvious this is the only program that works, but it's just not the right time for me."

Two years later, Marvin came back to start the program again. Marriage counseling had led him to divorce his verbally abusive wife, and there was a new woman in his life who loved him just the way he was. Marvin now had solely internal motivations for working with me again: he wanted to feel good about himself, and he wanted to be healthy. This is a classic case of the value of replacing external motivation tactics and strategies with internal motivation tactics and strategies.

As indicated above, the consultation interview is intended to determine if someone is a good candidate for the program. Another purpose of the initial consultation is to determine as accurately as possible if a client's ambivalence reflects justifiable feelings of hopelessness or what I refer to as an uncooperative personality profile. After years of applying the outcome data from my research, I'm almost invariably able to determine if someone is going to derive substantial benefit from the ICP. If I conclude someone is not a good candidate, I ask that person to consider that this might not be the right time, and I suggest waiting to begin the program until he or she can give it the priority that's needed. I'm completely comfortable saying, "This might not be the right time for you to start." It's much easier for me to make this suggestion if there's no fee attached at the front end.

MY ENCOUNTER WITH DEIDRE

I saw the flashing red light on my answering machine as soon as I opened my office door. Since it was a Monday, I surmised that the message was probably a query call from a potential client. Why? Calls from referrals are usually made over the weekend, because Monday seems to be the day when people are prepared to begin a diet regimen.

The message was from a woman named Deidre, who indicated that her close friend Melanie had given her my telephone number. Deidre left three phone numbers. She wanted to make sure that I returned her call. Leaving three numbers is a behavior that suggested a heightened degree of internal motivation and a strong measurement of commitment. I returned her call, and we made an appointment for the following Thursday at 3:00 p.m.

Though this next point may seem insignificant, I breathed a great sigh of relief when Deidre arrived for our appointment exactly on the dot. You'll soon come to appreciate how and why timeliness is one of the six behaviors that my research shows to have a highly significant statistical correlation to success during the first month and beyond.

Greeting me at the door is a pretty woman in her mid- to late thirties. She's about five feet four inches tall and weighs well over two hundred pounds. Her outfit is stylish, except for a large stain on her blouse. Her first words are an apology for her unkempt appearance. She tells me that on the way over, she had a small mishap while eating lunch, then explains, "I didn't want to be late or cancel our appointment, so I didn't go home to change my blouse."

We walk into my office. Bud, my Yorkshire terrier, demands that his new friend give him the attention he deserves. Deidre happily complies. His immediate needs satisfied, Bud retreats to his bed, which is located under my desk. This canine ritual seems to put people at ease, and, indeed, my initial goal is to help Deidre become relaxed and comfortable as soon as possible.

You see, there is a general anxiety associated with obesity. People who are overweight are highly visible, and, therefore, their weight issue is undeniable. Because of my own history, I understand more than most the shame and embarrassment of being overweight, so my task is to immediately create a safe and relaxed atmosphere.

Deidre is about to tell me her story. Not the superficial background information that's required pro forma by putative counselors employed in the dieting industry, but the real story that is the soul of her perennial weight-loss struggle. You know—the narrative and the personal and intimate details about why she made the call.

It's important to note that the unlicensed (and often untrained or marginally trained) counselors in many commercial diet programs are by law restricted in how they are allowed to respond when their customers divulge personal information. They're not permitted to posture as psychotherapists, analyze thoughts or feelings, nor interpret or speculate about their clients' underlying motivations for their behaviors. Most of these so-called weight-loss experts are really there to pitch the program and market the products associated with it.

In contrast, as a state-licensed clinical psychotherapist, it's my legal and ethical responsibility to help people analyze their motives and interpret their thoughts and feelings, while helping them uncover possible meanings for their behavior. I feel quite privileged when patients are ready to disclose the intimate details of their lifelong struggle with their weight.

I always begin the consultation interview with the same question: "What got you here?" This is the first face-to-face data-gathering moment for the purpose of hypothesizing whether the client will benefit from the ICP treatment protocol. I ask the question, then just sit back and listen.

Deidre begins by telling me that for more than twenty-five years, she'd tried virtually every conceivable diet and weight-loss program. She relates how the last diet had just about done her in. Deidre feels like a complete failure, convinced that her destiny of being fat had been preordained at birth. She says, "I made a decision that my dieting days were over. That was four years ago." Then she belatedly realized that her friend Melanie was gradually losing weight. Deidre says, "I hadn't paid much attention to it, because in the past she had lost weight, like me, only to gain it back, like me. But it had now been more than two years, and she's still keeping the weight off."

Deidre asked Melanie out to lunch and inquired about what diet Melanie was on. Melanie gave a look Deidre had never seen before. "She told me, nicely but firmly, that she was not on a diet. She went on to explain that it was hard to describe the process because of how personal the program is."

Melanie added, "I must admit that, at first, when I began the Immaculate Consumption Program, all I was interested in was that the scale continued to go down. I never believed that I'd be part of Dr. Solomon's documented 84 percent success rate, but slowly I began to realize that I was learning new eating habits. I was learning how to assert myself and make smart eating choices. I was investing time and money, and conforming to the personalized program that I created became my number-one priority. All I knew was that the mirror was my enemy, and I didn't want to end up ever again taking meds because of being overweight."

Melanie explained to Deidre that not getting her needs met was a big problem with all the other diets she had tried, but when she began implementing the ICP protocol, the contrast became obvious.

Deidre listened while her friend shared an incident that hit close to home. Melanie disclosed that she went to visit her mom several months after she began the program. She opened her mom's door only to get a familiar whiff of something baking in the oven. Knowing her daughter was coming for a visit, Melanie's mom had made her favorite cookies. "Mom knew I was trying to lose weight," Melanie said.

Then Melanie told Deidre, "A few moments later, Mom came out of the kitchen with a huge smile and placed a tray of warm cookies on the coffee table. I took the cookies from the table and placed them on the floor. I stood up and began jumping up and down, stomping them. I kissed Mom and left. Something happened when I stomped the cookies. It's as if I had assassinated the cookie monster that day, and I haven't looked back. That was a year ago, and Mom hasn't made me cookies since. There's one unexpected result: my mom and I have never been closer. Not only that, she asked for Dr. Solomon's number six months after the incident. Now, my mom's down twenty-five of the fifty pounds she wants to lose."

Deidre goes on to tell me, "Melanie handed me your card and told me the first visit is free. That was a year ago, and finally I'm here."

Deidre has given me some mixed messages. She wanted to meet with me, but I could sense that she didn't have any faith that she could succeed. I'm also curious why she had waited a year before calling me. My primary purpose for her consultation interview is to decipher these messages. Based on outcome data derived from my research, combined with three decades of clinical work, I had fine-tuned an assessment tool that would help me determine whether Deidre would benefit from the Immaculate Consumption Program.

I have learned how to draw out the true feelings and behaviors that motivate people to make the call for an initial appointment. The precipitating event serves as a behavioral and psychological template that defines people's embedded dieting mind-set. Failed ex-dieters invariably have feelings of embarrassment that must be brought to the surface and deactivated. The fail-safe way to manage feelings of dissonance, discouragement, and pessimism isn't to sublimate the reality of previous dieting setbacks but to acknowledge them by making them highly visible. The process of people disclosing their story reveals the baseline concepts that must be replaced with new concepts and experiences, which will result from adherence to the ICP protocol.

Keeping this in mind, I ask two questions: "What caused you to make the decision to call me?" and "Do you know the exact moment when you made the actual decision?" If someone retrieves and discloses the exact-moment incident for the decision, it indicates a capacity to be transparent.

Deidre reveals what had precipitated her call, and she indicates the exact moment she made the decision to call me. The precipitating event was something that happened the preceding Thursday, at 1:00 p.m.

"While window shopping," she says, "I leaned over to look at a handbag in the window. I wasn't prepared to see my reflection. At first, I didn't even realize who it was. Then, BAM, it was like someone just threw ice water in my face. Yes, it was *me*, and, in that instant, it felt like I had just awoken from a dream, or, in this case, a nightmare. The mirror image made it impossible for me to delude myself any longer. At that very moment, I realized that I desperately needed to call you and schedule an appointment, ASAP."

Deidre begins to cry and tells me that she had a confession to make. "Knowing that I was going to start a new diet, I stopped for my last meal," she said. "I ordered a burger, fries with ketchup, and a chocolate shake. Driving away from the take-out window, I accelerated too quickly. Fries and the chocolate shake spilled all over my blouse. At this moment, I'm feeling something I've never felt before about any previous diet. I'm certain that the only way this program can work is to be completely honest. I feel that I had to tell you the truth."

My task throughout this book is to encourage an atmosphere of positive reinforcement while attempting to minimize negative or aversive feelings from past weight-loss attempts. In Deidre's case, I achieve this by normalizing her last meal event.

To assuage Deidre's feelings of shame and embarrassment, I tell her that 99 percent of the clients I work with have a last meal before coming to the consultation interview. She is obviously relieved to learn this.

Deidre's confession is a perfect opportunity for me to explain the significant difference between the ICP and all other weight-loss methods: learning how to assume complete responsibility for one's eating decisions and behaviors. A "last meal" mind-set reflects the client's belief that all his or her favorite foods will have to be given up and that dieting represents the only way to lose weight. Indeed, submitting to the dieting rules of other programs had been the only way that Deidre knew how to lose weight. Weight loss is the shared goal of both the ICP and traditional dieting programs, but that's the only common denominator. I explain to Deidre that, unlike a diet, with its rigid constraints on what foods one is allowed and not allowed to eat, she does not have to give up all her favorite foods to lose weight with the ICP. Upon hearing this, she (like all my clients) gives me a look of disbelief.

I need to restore both Deidre's optimism and confidence, which has been extinguished as a consequence of her past weight-loss failures. I have always strongly believed it's in our nature to seek reasons for hope. Optimism is a powerful force that can mow down the mental and emotional states that can impede us from attaining our goals. Guilt, embarrassment, and shame were etched on Deidre's face when I first laid eyes on her. She needs to become convinced that she has finally met a professional who has the answers she has been searching for her entire life.

Deidre is about to be furnished with the final *raison d'être* for the consultation interview: hope. I want to bring her shame out into the open and have her conclude that she's now in the hands of a highly skilled expert who could lead her from the shadows of despair. I also want to restore her optimism that her weight-loss goals are actually attainable. Deidre's trust in the ICP and in me is imperative at the onset of the program, because it will serve as the bedrock for adherence to the treatment protocol I would subsequently introduce. I look into her eyes and say, "Deidre, it's time for you to sit back so I can give my spiel."

ESTABLISHING CREDIBILITY

After three decades of working in private practice, I've come to appreciate that one way to enhance a learning experience is to disclose personal information. I long ago discovered that potential clients became more receptive to hearing about the ICP protocol when they realized I, like them, had experienced dieting despair. The most effective method to make learning more likely to occur is for me to relate my personal weight-loss history.

My favorite part of the consultation interview is about to begin. I reach over to pick up the folder on my desk, then remove my "before" photo and hand it to Deidre. Even after all these years, I still get a kick out of the "Oh, this can't be you" reaction. Deidre doesn't disappoint me.

Studying the picture intently, she comments, "Well, it's the same nose, eyes, and hair color, but I still can't believe it's you."

"Yes," I tell her, "that's me in 1977 at two hundred twenty pounds. I've kept off over seventy pounds since 1980."

While she is studying the picture, I disclose that my weight-loss journey began with diet pills (amphetamines) when I was ten years old and that during the following twenty years my weight would fluctuate between twenty to sixty pounds every year, depending on what diet I was on and whether I could score diet pills. I told Deidre, "In 1968, I decided to stop the pills. Slowly, over the years, I ballooned to two hundred twenty pounds. I attribute my own weight-loss success to the very same principles I'll be discussing with you. This is the only system that has ever worked for me to keep weight off. My journey spinning around on the dieting carousel finally stopped in 1980."

Deidre's eyes slowly and steadily begin to look up from the picture. She just smiles.

If you want to develop complete responsibility for your eating decisions and behaviors, learn and implement the two scientific principles conveyed in the following chapters. The fact of the matter is that learning and implementing both principles must become the top priority in your life, for one month at a minimum.

3

◆

LAYING THE FOUNDATION
FOR SELF-ACTUALIZATION

Deidre's consultation interview is coming to a close. The consultation has provided me with a great deal of information, and it is now time for Deidre to determine if she is ready and willing to start the Immaculate Consumption Program.

It is important to give Deidre the option to say yes or no without exerting any pressure. I suggest that she consider calling other clients with whom I had worked and/or those currently in different stages of the program. (I had secured confidentiality releases permitting these contacts.) Information provided by these clients would help Deidre make an informed decision. I assure her that I'd been practicing for decades and that if she decides not to start the program and subsequently changes her mind, I would be available at a later time.

Smiling as she handed back my picture, Deidre looks me straight in the eyes and says, "There is no need for me to think about what I want to do." She begins to cry and says, "It feels like you have a real handle on this. In light of your own obviously successful battle with weight, I feel a sense of hope that I've never felt before, and I'm ready to start as soon as possible.

"When can I start?"

I open up my date book and tell her, "A week from today."

Deidre says, "I'd rather not wait; don't you have anything sooner?"

My answer is a decisive "No."

Deidre has the look of a deer in the headlights. A moment later, she says, "I woke up this morning prepared to begin losing my weight, so I was ready to do whatever you told me to do. It sounds like your program is the answer I've been looking for my whole life, and now you're asking me to wait?"

It's important to acknowledge that failed ex-dieters are prone to repeat patterns they've previously learned. Deidre's patterns resulted from having been inculcated with rigid attitudes about dieting. Because of her past disappointments, the potential for failing again weighed heavily on her shoulders. Deidre's fears seemed warranted. She believed that not losing weight immediately would cause her motivation to waver. While her fears appeared reasonable, she needed to realize how unjustified they actually were.

REFLECTION ENCOURAGES SELF-DISCOVERY

Virtually every person following a dieting program simply accepts the necessity for blindly obeying the rules designed by the supposed gurus who developed that program. The result of this regimented obedience was plainly evident in Deidre's embedded mind-set. When she first walked into my office, Deidre's independent thinking had already been replaced with a willingness to be led in directions that had been determined, or at least strongly influenced, by the thinking of others.

Mandatory compliance with externally imposed rules is the primary feature that creates a dieter's resistance and rebelliousness at those critical junctures when it ultimately becomes impossible for the dieter to follow the rules. A noncompliant event has a near 100 percent probability of occurring in virtually every dieting program. A dieter will typically perceive such an event as a failure, which weighs heavily on the dieter's emotional well-being. As a result, the dieter develops a commonly held belief system about the failure: if only he or she had had the willpower to scrupulously follow the dieting rules, the diet would have succeeded.

Deidre always did what she was told, until she finally hit the wall of noncompliance. With every diet she tried, she came to a point where compliance with external rules became impossible for her. Then she would lament that if only she had the resolve to obey the food rules, she would have undoubtedly succeeded. In effect, Deidre laid a major guilt trip on herself. Ipso facto, she concluded that failing to lose weight was all her fault. After sufficient time spent emotionally rebounding, she would begin yet another diet and repeat the cycle of compliance with the rules, until, once again, she reached the point of noncompliance.

Given her dieting history, it felt unnatural and stress inducing to delay—for even one week—establishing a disciplined regimen for attaining her long-term weight-loss goal. My admonition that she wait seemed patently unreasonable. Deidre felt as if she was being set up for failure by my request that she be nonadherent to seemingly commonsense traditional dieting strictures, just as she was about to begin the ICP and her enthusiasm was at its peak.

Reliance on others for the nuts and bolts of what's required to lose weight removes the dieters' opportunity to rely on their own firsthand observations and experiences. Skills for taking personal responsibility for choices are poorly developed or simply disregarded. After all, the dieting industry relies on repeat consumers; teaching dieters to take personal responsibility is counterproductive to the industry's extraordinarily profitable business model.

Deidre's reaction to the one-week hiatus signaled that, on both a conscious and unconscious level, she felt she had to comply with a rule that was embossed in her mind, namely: to maximize the effect of your current motivation and willpower, you must not defer or delay implementing the program that will immediately begin helping you attain your weight-loss goal. Every diet Deidre had tried—and there had been many—conditioned her to believe that success was contingent upon obeying external commandments, getting a running start, and instantly capitalizing on her new-found enthusiasm. Given this doctrinaire mind-set, it seemed perfectly natural for her to want to start complying with the "new ICP rules" as soon as possible. This explains why virtually all clients who perceive themselves as failed dieters initially have minimal trust in themselves and absolute trust in me.

The ultimate goal of the ICP protocol is to help people develop skills and habits that enable them to take personal responsibility for their eating behaviors. Before the ICP research methodology can begin, however, clients must first be cognizant of their current food-related behaviors; in other words, they must identify their baseline behaviors. For this reason, I counsel my clients to do two things during the week between the consultation interview and the intake session:

1. Keep all your current eating behaviors *stable and unchanged.*
2. Stay off the scale.

These admonitions allow clients to develop independent thinking skills and to ponder their preconceived ideas about what constitutes the most rational initial strategy for losing weight. The recommendations also alleviate the stress of being forced to comply, from the get-go, with externally imposed rules—particularly with regard to eating. Ideally, following these precepts will encourage clients to begin viewing and assessing their current behaviors more dispassionately, and by so doing, to be more able to evaluate with added objectivity their future food-related experiences. In turn, this introspection will help clients better manage the negative feelings associated with the inevitable days of overconsumption. The waiting period is thus an exercise in temporarily holding in abeyance goal-obsessive habits and replacing them with more rational and realistic behaviors that will facilitate long-term weight loss and successful weight management.

Imagine that you attend a lecture to hear about a method offering weight reduction and permanent management of the weight lost. As the lecturer arrives at the podium, she is holding a box and says, "What's inside this box is the one and only answer for lifelong control of eating behaviors before, during, and after the moment of consumption. Here's my guarantee: your cure for being overweight will be found inside this box." The lecturer continues, "I'm offering that box to you right now. If you decide to open up the lid and peer in, you'll come face to face with a mirror."

The message is obvious: you are the only one able to provide the solutions you're looking for when it comes to a successful weight-loss experience. Now, it's one thing to look at the mirror. It's an entirely different occurrence, and one that requires effort, to actually *see* the image that is reflected back.

The waiting period is the first step in helping you determine solutions

for lifelong control of eating behaviors based on your own firsthand observations and experiences. In order to develop the skills necessary to change
your eating behaviors and habits, you must first establish a baseline for your
current eating behaviors and habits. The start of the waiting period begins
the *experiential* phase of your weight-loss journey.

ENHANCING YOUR PROBLEM-SOLVING SKILLS

Rather than a "one size fits all" methodology that is characteristic of the
typical mass-marketed diet programs, the ICP emphasizes learning how to
customize weight-loss and weight-loss maintenance strategies with an individualized eating plan *that works best for you.*

To address and assuage her anxiety and stress about having to wait a
week before the next visit, I explain to Deidre that, in this program, she will
become a single-subject researcher (i.e., she'll be both the researcher and
the research subject, as more fully explained in the following chapters). I
go on to tell her that learning involves taking an action and reflecting upon
the results—*your own results.* This leads to the acquisition of more effective
problem-solving skills. Through systematic application of the ICP methodology, she will take an action and then assess the results to determine what
works best for her.

I could see that Deidre revels in the fact that she would generate her
own rules based upon the results of her own systematic research. In her past
dieting attempts, she always came to a point where obedience to external
rules became unmanageable and led to her so-called failure on the diet.
She comments, "Just like you said, this is going to be my experiment. I
especially like the fact that my role is going to be that of a single-subject
researcher and that the laboratory for my personal experiment will be my
own life."

I explain that getting away from goal achievement–type habits for one
week certainly would not force her to abandon successful techniques that
have worked in the past; however, making current behaviors visible and
analyzing the flaws in those behaviors would help her jettison and unlearn
what hasn't worked in the past so that she can develop and learn behaviors
that will work more successfully in the future.

I proceed to explain to Deidre that if she follows this objective assessment precept, it will result in improving her ability to analyze her eating behaviors more dispassionately and, therefore, more objectively. The result is a *de-emotionalizing effect* that brings current behaviors out in the open. The visibility of current eating behaviors sets the stage for a journey of *self-exploration* that is a core element of the ICP method. The one-week hiatus from dieting between the consultation interview and the intake session is in preparation for developing three qualities that comprise the profile of those capable of self-management. These include acquiring skills in the following areas:

1. Self-evaluation.

2. Self-intervention.

3. Problem-solving.

I tell Deidre that:

- The ICP will provide you with a methodology to expand on and hone these qualities and actualize your ability to lose weight and maintain your weight loss.

- You'll come to appreciate that you're no different than other people who experience body-weight fluctuations.

- You'll also come to realize that it's okay to lose, gain, and maintain weight within what are generally considered to be *normal ranges*.

- You will determine for yourself what your normal weight range should be, and you will use the insights you'll acquire about yourself through your subsequent research to guide your food choices and regulate your behaviors.

- The process will be internally motivated, not externally dictated.

- The self-management skills you will cultivate through the ICP will help you attain self-actualization-type strategies for losing weight and maintaining your weight loss.

ENDING THE CONSULTATION INTERVIEW WITH DEIDRE

We are ready to end the consultation interview when Deidre finally asks the expected million-dollar question: "If I have to wait a week, what am I supposed to do until then?" As usual, my answer is firm: "*Nothing.*" Then I say, in a reassuring tone, "At this time, don't change anything."

I inform Deidre that putting off the start of the program for a week could be the hardest part of the program and that I receive the most frequent complaints from clients about this aspect. I also acknowledge that the no-rules week might be a bit anxiety provoking at first. But I assure Deidre that she isn't going on a diet where all her favorite foods would be taken away. No one is going to tell her what should or shouldn't be eaten. I again remind Deidre: "Do what you would normally do. Try not to diet, and remember to stay off the scale."

As indicated previously, these suggestions are in complete opposition to what dieters expect during the days leading up to the start of a diet. Staying off the scale for the first week is very hard, but it is one of the most import-ant admonitions. The scale has always provided the indisputable measure-ment of weight-loss outcome, and dieters can become very reliant on it. The weighing-in procedure each morning is addicting. Though staying off the scale for a week can be extremely challenging, it has proven to be one of the most important indicators of a successful outcome in the ICP before the experiment or treatment phase begins.

Deidre looks me straight in the eyes and says, "I've never felt this way before. I just know that this is going to work." Then she says, "I realize that I have to wait a week before I start the program. This is the first time that I'm thinking into the future about losing weight. The sense of immediacy I've always felt is gone. Also, I somehow don't have feelings of being as desperate as I have been every other time I started a new diet."

Having reached the end the of the consultation interview, we head for the door.

4

♦

THE DOWNSIDE OF LINKING EXERCISE TO WEIGHT LOSS

Deidre's ingrained preconceptions about dieting—which included strictly obeying food rules and exercising to lose weight—became evident as soon as the consultation interview ended. As we head for the door, she says, "I'm so excited. On the way home there's a gym down the block from my house, and I intend to join today—in fact, right now!" I ask her if she'd ever been to a gym. She responds, "No."

It is imperative that I drive home the point I am about to make. Taking a deep breath, I tell her, "Do not, for any reason, begin an exercise program at this time."

She looks at me in disbelief, as if I am an alien from another planet, and replies, "I've never heard advice like this before." As she looks at me in disbelief, all I say is, "Trust me." Deidre responds that she would.

She then proceeds to say exactly what the majority of my patients say: "Actually, I feel a tremendous sense of relief about not having to exercise. I'm confused, but I feel that a tremendous weight has been taken off my shoulders." Deidre leaves smiling and gently nodding her head up and down. She walks out the door and says, "Thank you."

MANAGING EXPECTANCY BELIEFS

All dieters are prone to rely on and repeat ad nauseam the behavior patterns they believe will determine the success of the diet they choose, even if these patterns have proven unsuccessful in the past. These reiterations coalesce into a series of ritualistic procedures established from the onset of all weight-loss methods—a supposedly tailored and personalized equation about how the dieter's goal-weight expectations will ideally be realized. The following phrase identifies one of the most prevalent common denominators that often doom the long-term success of a dieting program: *the initial pairing of exercise with weight loss.* Indeed, most diet "experts" share an almost sacred conviction that the only way to attain weight-loss success is by strict adherence to a set of duly sanctioned, well established, and externally imposed litany of rules that invariably includes exercise.

The National Weight Control Registry (NWCR), which was founded in 1994, is considered the most influential gold standard in the weight-loss field. This registry has supplied the largest amount of research data about long-term weight loss and weight-loss maintenance in the United States. The goal of the NWCR project was to collect information in an attempt to identify, investigate the characteristics of, and profile those who succeeded at long-term weight loss. The study was comprised of a detailed questionnaire mailed to those who claimed to fit the study's population—dieters who attained long-term weight-loss success. Annual follow-up questionnaires were subsequently mailed to the same people.

To date, this registry has tracked over ten thousand participants who have lost a significant amount of weight and kept it off for at least seven years. The self-reporting data supplied by the people who signed up for the study is quite revealing. Ninety-eight percent of participants modified decisions about their food choices, and 90 percent relied upon exercise for their weight-management goals. As a result of the study, two overarching rules emerged about which everyone in the weight-loss industry agreed: *eat less and exercise more.*

Not all people are candidates for externally imposed exercise regimes that are grafted onto their dieting programs from the beginning, and when they fall off the exercise wagon, they may also fall off other elements of the diet-plan wagon. In contrast, the Immaculate Consumption Program lets clients decide if and when they want to begin exercising, and that's the salient point! In my opinion, if there is a failing in the NWCR research, it is that researchers didn't study data from the modus operandi of the unsuccessful weight-loss population for the purposes of comparing and identifying the point when their attempts at dieting began to fail. In other words, they didn't compile data from unsuccessful dieters about the juncture where the dieters abandoned their self-control. Was an externally imposed dieting regime the primary culprit? What effect did an externally imposed exercise regime have on their dieting failures?

Currently, the NWCR study has contributed to suppositions that sustained weight-loss success will be achieved when dieters adhere to a basic formula of *convincing indicators* (CIs). After a twenty-year analysis of the data, the registry detected five major behaviors of people with long-term weight-loss maintenance—convincing indicators—and concluded that a person can maintain successful weight loss by following the following guidelines, the five CIs:

1. Modify their food intake (98 percent did so).
2. Eat breakfast every day (78 percent did so).
3. Weigh themselves at least once a week (75 percent did so).
4. Watch less than ten hours of TV per week (62 percent did so).
5. Exercise, on average, one hour per day (90 percent did so).

All weight-loss programs are based on the primary CI of modifying food intake, and most, if not all, include the CI of exercise as part of the weight-loss protocol. Since all weight-loss methods are tarred with the same brush, Deidre's look of bewilderment when I told her not to begin an exercise routine was based on the precepts advocated by the other programs she had tried. As such, her confusion was understandable.

The insistence that an exercise program is the primary contributing factor for long-term weight-loss success, while appearing reasonable, is in reality the result of faulty reasoning. It will become clear why and how the results of the NWCR study can actually lead many dieters to draw flawed conclusions that may work at cross-purposes with attaining and sustaining their weight-loss goals.

The fact is that exercise should never be relied upon either to lose weight or to maintain weight loss. *To be effective over the long term, an exercise regime should be voluntary and not externally imposed.* After more than three decades of working with patients, it's become clear to me that imposing an exercise routine is not a causal factor in achieving successful and sustained weight loss. Exercise does not help people develop new strategies and habits for making their food choices. But when people who apply the ICP protocol experience successful and sustainable weight reduction, they begin to acquire confidence in their ability to retain their weight loss by modifying their behaviors and making more astute food choices. These people then often make a deliberate (and voluntary) choice to exercise as a way to take better care of themselves, not as a way to lose weight or maintain their weight loss.

I CAN EXERCISE AWAY THE CALORIC EVIDENCE

If you remember, Melanie was the person who referred Deidre to me. Melanie's story will help you appreciate why you should never comply with weight-loss rules that experts in the dieting industry have deemed necessary for successful dieting and weight management, and especially those that link exercise with a food-consumption regimen for the purpose of weight management. Let's take a closer look at Melanie's dieting history.

Melanie came to see me in the early 1990s. She had begun her last diet more than two years previously. It was a highly restrictive food program, and it was one of the most dramatic examples of what I call the "fast and furious" approach to losing weight.

Such approaches especially appeal to a population of dieters who have inexhaustible physical energy, enthusiasm, and a high strive-to-achieve quotient. I categorize this population as the "Holy Moly! I'm on top of the world. I can accomplish anything!" group; it's a population that possesses a "nothing can deter me" mind-set about losing weight. It may sound as if those who fit into this group are a bit manic, and in many cases they certainly verge on being so.

Though perhaps not to this magnified extent, many dieters are predisposed to exaggerated feelings of eagerness and passion about establishing weight-loss goals at the onset of every diet. This goal-achievement attitude is beneficial because it reinforces compliance and adherence to whatever the dieting protocols require.

Melanie was certainly in a group that I categorize as highly motivated dieters. Those who are best described by this category are inclined to exhibit overachievement-type behaviors. They fervently adhere to the strict rules prescribed by their dieting protocols, which typically impose significant restrictions on food intake and a rigorous special-forces style of exercise.

Physical activities thus become intrinsically linked with the diet as a primary means to burn calories and lose weight more effectively. In conjunction with the diet's restricted food intake, the pleasurable effects of exercise and the likely associated release of endorphins team up to produce dramatic weight loss. This seals the deal for this driven population of dieters. It's a formula that works for some in the short term and for a very few (especially those who are naturally predisposed to exercise) in the long term.

Melanie's "Delta Force-like" exercise regimen included two-hour gym workouts four days per week, translating into her working out every other day. On her gym days, she'd get up at 5:00 a.m. during the week and a little later on Saturdays. Sunday was always her day off from the gym. On her three gym days off, she would typically get together with friends after work on the weekdays and during the midmorning on Sunday for some kind of physical activity, such as tennis, hiking in the park, jogging, swimming, or inline skating.

Melanie saw a rapid weight loss and dropped close to twenty-five pounds in a little over three months. At the end of three months, more food options were introduced. These were good, safe, and healthy foods. Several weeks into this stage, it happened: she saw the television commercial.

Melanie hadn't seen this commercial before. She watched intently while the good-looking young actor set a white cardboard box down on his coffee table. As he opened the box, steam wafted into the air. Melanie swore the aroma had actually seeped into her living room. Slowly lifting a slice of piping-hot pizza, melting with cheese, he took the first bite. His face reflected pure ecstasy.

Melanie's reaction was visceral. Then her self-talk started: "Mmm. Wow, that pizza looks amazing. Stop it! I remember how good pizza tasted. *Stop*! Are you crazy? You know how you'll feel afterward! But I want it. Can eating two slices of pizza possibly hurt? After all, it's a normal dinner for most people. Quick, go look at your fat picture on the fridge! But I've been so good. I deserve it."

Melanie felt herself succumbing to temptation, and that was the moment she made the deal with the devil. She was able to deflect the consequence of her pizza-consuming behavior by resorting to a convenient rationalization: "OK, I'll order the pizza this one time, because I can just go to the track tomorrow and jog an extra eight miles." At the exact permission-giving moment, the sense of relief she felt from that rationalization evoked another conniving rationalization: "If I'm clever, I can get away with it."

Such justifications will work for a few moments or perhaps a few days, but ultimately one's self-deception shatters, and the justifications won't work anymore. More and more lapses will occur, and more and more justifications will have to be initiated to counteract the overconsumption. All order will begin to crumble in the dieter's world, and the pieces will no longer fit together.

The major contributing factor for why Melanie's diet had begun its inexorable downward slide stemmed from her initial rationalization to cheat "this one time" by promising herself that she'd exercise more vigorously tomorrow. It's a self-delusional mind-set that hinges on being able to repay the piper down the road. This is the quintessential common denominator of all such excuses and rationalizations for flawed food choices that attempt to deny cause-and-effect realities and responsibility for one's actions. This may sound harsh, but the slide is inextricably linked to the attempt to follow a relentless, externally imposed, and unforgiving dieting regimen. Simply stated, once you break the rules and fall off the wagon, it's hard to get back on the wagon. Your self-control, willpower, drive, and determination suddenly and inexorably evaporate.

In an effort to rid herself of anxiety, Melanie did what most people do when relying heavily on exercise for weight management. They justify subsequent transgressions by rationalizing, "I can always burn off the caloric evidence by exercising more." Melanie succumbed to her craving, picked up the phone, and pressed the speed-dial button for the pizza joint. The special meat lover's loaded pizza was delivered and devoured in less than forty-five minutes.

A decision to use exercise as a justification to overeat or to break the rules is usually the first deviation from the dieting program's food dictates. An unrecoverable relapse occurs, because the rationalization to rely on exercise to atone for poor food choices simply deflects the consequences of the counterproductive eating behaviors. Deciding to exercise to offset the caloric evidence provides a superficial, but seemingly logical and reasonable, solution for the forbidden-food escapade but is typically a prelude to a series of other forbidden-food escapades.

For Melanie, the unrecoverable relapse required only one behavior that dredged up all her old feelings of personal failure, frustration, and disappointment. This time it was a Pizza Temptation (analogous to Deidre's Pink Box Temptation) that threatened to reignite the familiar array of self-sabotaging food habits and choices that would spread like a raging forest fire and once again potentially engulf her life.

Unfortunately, virtually every dieter will, at some point, come face to face with this kind of momentous decision; that is, a decision of whether to break the food rules and thereby risk an unrecoverable relapse. A craving response forces a key decision-making moment when two opposing desires are evoked at the same time. These desires consist of a positive, goal-oriented choice that supports weight-loss success versus a negative, counterproductive submission to deleterious food cravings. The second option clearly conflicts with the first. In this situation, the internal brat is whining, "I want what I want when I want it, and I want it now!" The first one or two craving episodes can sometimes be handled successfully, but, eventually, satisfying the demands for immediate gratification of the craving responses will typically prevail.

The first nonadherence to the externally imposed dictates of the diet is the moment of truth (e.g., a Pizza or Pink Box Moment), and most often, it is all that is needed to initiate an unrecoverable relapse. If exercise is associated with weight-loss success, nonadherence to the exercise regimen can act as the first gateway that opens up the floodgates to other indiscretions.

MAKING YOUR BODY AN ALLY

It bears repeated emphasis that *exercise should never be relied upon either to lose weight or to retain weight loss.* Many of my clients do decide to introduce exercise into their weekly schedule after they have developed their weight-loss and weight-management skills, but that decision is not dictated by the ICP protocol. Cindy's story exemplifies this point.

Cindy met with me three years after her last dieting experience. Within the first few weeks of starting the program, she became more and more confident in her ability to manage incidents that were previously considered breaking the rules. As Cindy progressed through the program, she recognized how her food rules had evolved from being externally dictated by a diet to being internally dictated by her own, individual ICP protocol. She was learning how to create her own food rules that were congruent with her experiences, expectations, and mental attitudes.

On her previous diets, any stressful event would, in all probability, trigger an unrecoverable relapse. But now, Cindy was dealing with stressors more effectively. Rather than relying on food as her only coping strategy, she was learning a vast array of other strategies, besides eating, to self-soothe.

In all her past weight-loss attempts, Cindy had been forced to invoke the same protocol for her food consumption that was used for dealing with all addictive substances, a protocol predicated on relapse-prevention strategies. As is the case for heroin addiction, banned foods must be completely avoided, and it is vital to do everything to prevent their reintroduction. Relying on the medical model for treating addiction, traditional diets place foods considered bad for you in the same category as heroin or other addictive substances. This model equates flawed food choices and eating behavior with a reversion to a diseased state.

There is one obvious problem with doing this: We can survive without heroin, but without food, we'll die. Resorting to the medical model that advocates total abstinence erroneously equates the willpower to resist deleterious drugs or alcohol with the willpower to resist high-calorie foods. This dooms dieters to relapses and all-but-certain failure over the long run.

Cindy was beginning to realize that deviations from goal-directed weight-loss behaviors would inevitably occur. Rather than focusing on relapse prevention, which requires abstinence, she was able to recognize that occasional reversions, regressions, and deviations were not only predictable, but they were actually normal. This represented a major shift in her thinking and resulted in a significant reduction in her angst and guilt about sporadically breaking her own food rules.

I'd been working with Cindy for about a year, during which time she had lost approximately fifty pounds. She came in one day and relayed an incident that had occurred the previous evening. A phone call from her mother had left Cindy feeling anxious. She decided it would be a good time to get some fresh air, so she put the leash on her dog for his usual walk around the block. While walking, she looked across the street and noticed a woman with a dog similar to hers going into the neighborhood park.

It was fall, Cindy's favorite time of year. This motivated her to go on a longer walk than usual, and she decided to deviate from her usual routine and explore the neighborhood park instead. Halfway through, she noticed some people in an exercise area located in the far corner of the park. They appeared to be using some kind of stationary apparatus. Wandering over, she found herself in front of a step that was about two feet high. Cautiously at first, she stepped up and then down, using her right foot and then her left. Before long, she had completed a set of ten step-ups. At that moment, Cindy's decision to move her body and perform the exercise had nothing to do with a motivation to achieve her weight-loss goal. It derived more from curiosity.

Cindy talked about how, in the past, disturbing calls from her mother would have caused a self-soothing event with food. This time, however, she made a decision to go for an extended walk and somehow ended up in the exercise area of her neighborhood park. Cindy explained that her anxiety disappeared after completing the set of ten step-ups. She spoke about a tremendous sense of accomplishment from not turning to food in response to her mother's call. And she shared that, after completing the ten step-ups, she felt a sense of well-being she'd never experienced before.

Cindy's response to her mother's call was directly linked to her learning curve and confirmed that her newfound self-determined actions resulted from a burgeoning and more independently oriented mind-set (in contrast to her previously more robotic and acquiescent mind-set). The effect is a conscious cognitive shift in thinking about the factors that can contribute significantly to enhanced weight loss, healthier food behaviors and choices, and improved weight-loss management. In the process, the negative physical and emotional effects of previous dieting failures were also neu-tralized. These elements are deliberately targeted benchmarks of the ICP methodology.

I realized that it would require time for Cindy to turn completely

away from her historic dieting beliefs. For more than a year, she continued to hold onto some ingrained habits and attitudes that persisted from
her past negative dieting experiences. Unknowingly, she had been subjected
to dieting methods that had evolved from the medical model of disease,
in which overeating was seen as an illness that must be cured. Stereotypi-
cally, health providers are expected to possess all the skills and knowledge
needed to achieve this cure, and therefore, the patients' role in the traditional doctor/patient relationship is to be passive and dependent upon these
experts.

Cindy's need to resort to food as a coping strategy for her anxiety was
becoming less and less frequent since she had learned how to counteract
her previous self-defeating types of eating behaviors. As a result, her confidence about her food-management skills was skyrocketing. She told me,
"Without a question of doubt, my dieting days are over."

Still, submitting to rules was the only way Cindy knew how to be successful with losing weight. After she had described what transpired the day
before in the exercise area of the park, she said, "You told me I shouldn't
exercise. This is the longest I've ever stuck with any program. For the
first time in my life, I'm feeling a sense of permanence about my ability
to manage my weight loss. I don't want to do anything that will compromise my success." Cindy clearly was conflicted. She indicated her concern
when she tentatively asked, "Do you think it's okay if I go back to the park
and continue doing the steps?" I was smiling inside. "Of course," I replied.
"Obviously, you're exercising because *you* truly want to exercise and not to
lose weight. That's great!"

Cindy's desire to introduce exercise felt like nonadherence to a rule that
was set down at the onset of the program, and she didn't want to do anything
that would negatively affect her success. Hence, she was concerned. Yet
Cindy was learning how to take greater personal proactive responsibility for
her relationship with food.

The fact that Cindy even considered going against the rules indicated
that she was beginning to deconstruct her erroneous preconceptions about
what it takes to lose weight; she didn't have to submit to orders! This indicated her developing capacity for toppling her previously embedded belief
systems. She was personally assessing what goal achievement actually meant

to her. At the top of Cindy's list was researching alternatives to self-soothing with food. She was learning new coping strategies. Moving her body felt good. She was using exercise to de-stress, she had more energy, and she was beginning to see a toned body she never could have imagined. This represented the most self-directed and internally driven means for attaining her objectives. If this meant implementing an exercise regimen when it felt right to do so, then all the better!

Forming permanent, more beneficial habits derives from the ability to distill and learn from personal experiences, as opposed to being told what to do. True changes occur through exposure to information in a way that allows each person to research, assess, and pursue the appropriate individualized direction to follow. By deliberately creating this kind of personal discovery context, the opportunity for self-organized learning is made possible. Only then will one have the capacity for viewing personally acquired data as constructed and reconstructed by one's own interaction with the environment.

The most effective way to teach responsibility is to create and nurture constructive attitudes so that positive associations regarding taking responsibility and learning can occur. In 1969, Carl Rogers, a towering figure in the field of psychology, spoke about "self-organized" learning, stating that "enabling others *to learn to learn* is usually misconstrued as instructing them how to successfully submit to being taught."

Learning how to learn is addressed throughout the following chapters. This segue begins your journey of learning how to determine weight-loss and weight-maintenance behaviors that are right for you—and only you. You will discover that the only strategy for guaranteeing permanent habit formations is for you to develop your own self-directed behaviors.

5

◆

CLEANING OUT THE COBWEBS

Instinctively realizing when it's time to move on from what was once a strategically placed and highly functional trap for capturing its prey, the spider finally abandons its lair to seek a more promising location. It leaves behind deserted cobwebs amid the dust and lint that reside in the more inaccessible corners of our otherwise pristine closets and attics.

"Cleaning out the cobwebs" is the metaphor I have chosen for the title of this chapter, in which I describe how to skillfully handle the dieting cobwebs. This is the gradual letting-go phase of the Immaculate Consumption Program. This phase entails the long-overdue clearing out of the accumulated and often ineffectual weight-loss attitudes, beliefs, and behaviors that may have been cluttering your mind for decades.

CONFIRMATION BIAS CREATES
A STRANGLEHOLD ON DIETING BELIEFS

Everyone's way of thinking about the many mundane issues in life consists mainly of ingrained, subliminal habits and reactions. In countless instances, our thoughts, attitudes, and behaviors have become so automatic that they're often below our conscious level of awareness. Thus, our current system of beliefs is contingent upon thinking patterns derived from how our life experiences have programmed us to perceive and respond to the world around us.

People interpret and recall information very selectively. This is a specialized kind of thinking that reflects an amalgam of our existing attitudes. Our propensity to selectively view information about familiar situations enables us to automatically respond in routine or habitual ways. For example, you return from work and find dirty dishes on the kitchen table and immediately blame your teenage son for not putting them in the dishwasher as he has been repeatedly instructed. We thus continually interface with the world around us through the interplay of the past and the present. This reasoning process creates links in an embedded chain that causes us to act in a manner consistent with our belief system and experiences. Similar events occurring in our lives become bound with our thoughts, attitudes, and behaviors; that is, prior states determine later states. The scientific term for this process is *confirmation bias.*

Confirmation bias is a concept based upon research that has yielded four well-established principles of behavioral psychology, and it elucidates how:

1. Ideas are learned from and supported by previous experiences.

2. Personal opinions and conclusions are derived from fixed patterns of thoughts secured in our memory banks.

3. There is a biased preference for attitudes that confirm our preconceptions and expectations, whereas there is a biased dislike for attitudes that conflict with our preconceptions and expectations.

4. Existing attitudes persist because people interpret and recall experiences in a very discriminatory way and are attracted to information that supports their already intact belief system.

Confirmation bias is especially relevant in dieting. It is an established fact that past dieting experiences determine your current ways of thinking. And it is also an established fact that biases are supported by an essentially intact belief system at the onset of virtually all newly implemented weight-loss procedures. Weight-loss thinking patterns that share many common denominators are pervasive and represent what I refer to as one's personal dieting belief system. Dieters typically persist in holding onto these frequently counterproductive beliefs because they may have initially attained a modicum of weight-loss success using them in the short term, and confirmation bias has programmed them to disregard evidence showing that they have failed to maintain their weight loss in the long term.

Archived events—and particularly the maladaptive ones—often create a stranglehold on your current thoughts, feelings, and behaviors, and, by so doing, they can (to the experienced eye of the professionally trained clinician) reveal your personal dieting profile. One's ingrained dieting mentality may be so firmly fixed that changing directions can prove challenging and even psychologically threatening.

Most repeat dieters have been programmed to think and behave in certain ways. As previously mentioned, diets are based on the medical model of disease and have two common denominators:

1. A diet's food rules are externally imposed.

2. The dieter's adherence or nonadherence to these food rules is predictive of whether he or she will lose weight.

In traditional mass-marketed dieting programs, despite their supposed ostensible differences, the core medical model for weight management they all rely on forces the consumer to choose one quintessential course of action. Being limited to an externally imposed basic modus operandi squashes free will. Control of and responsibility for our actions is taken away from us, and we become willing, robotic participants in this mind-numbing process. Yet in the vast majority of cases, this mind-set ironically forms the basis of our entire dieting belief system.

Offering an alternative methodology and insights might be perceived as obliging dieters to relinquish their familiar dieting belief system, which may trigger knee-jerk defensiveness and resistance. When exposed to information inconsistent with prior beliefs, dieters often experience mental stress and emotional discomfort. They believe that if they dare deviate significantly in their current weight-loss attempts from their previous way of thinking and behaving, their efforts will somehow be jinxed and a priori produce negative consequences.

There is an obvious paradox in this mind-set: a belief on many dieters' part—whether consciously acknowledged or not—that because their previous experiences have repeatedly produced negative consequences in the short term or long term, their current contemplated course corrections are ultimately also destined to be futile. This transference phenomenon can generate a great deal of *anticipatory anxiety* when dieters are considering making risky changes in their weight-loss procedures.

After three decades spent poring over accumulated research data, I've come to appreciate that the typical weight-loss client with whom I interface is rarely capable of being immediately receptive to assimilating new perspectives, methods, and procedures. When heavily invested in one position and then confronted with another that disconfirms proven evidence (i.e., previous weight-loss failures or temporary successes), there's a natural inclination to go to great lengths to justify maintaining existing beliefs. The stranglehold of their *confirmation bias* is, at least initially, simply too powerful.

Dieters confronted with information inconsistent with their current belief system may experience an emotional state called *cognitive dissonance.* This state arises when they hold contradictory beliefs, and it can cause chaotic feelings and emotional discomfort. One the one hand, is the belief system that people must follow the dictates of a diet's food rules; on the other, is a program (the ICP) that will lead them to creating their own rules. Challenging a dieting belief system may create doubt and lead to resistance to the new incoming information. The result is noncompliant-type thoughts and behaviors, which must be prevented at all costs.

REMOVING THE STRANGLEHOLD

Because it is unrealistic to think you'll be capable of reversing your embedded dieting belief system at this juncture in the ICP, keeping cognitive dissonance at bay is the number-one priority. In so doing, resistance is defused and cooperation is enhanced as a prelude to subsequently introducing the actual treatment phase of the program. The key is to make the transition from the previous dieting regimes to the ICP protocol as seamless, nonthreatening, and effortless as possible. The guiding principle is: when clients aren't surprised or overwhelmed by new concepts, their defensiveness is reduced, and their receptivity to adapt to change is increased.

It may be helpful to view the process of transitioning from your previous dieting regimes to the novel ICP methodology offered in this book as a systematic bridge-building exercise. On one side of the bridge is your intact dieting belief system, which in all likelihood is based on the medical model of disease that views overeating as an illness that must be cured. On the other side of the bridge is the ICP method. In contrast to insisting that you subject yourself to rigid, externally imposed food rules, the ICP takes a different approach. Advancement toward the goals of weight loss and weight-loss sustainability necessitates that you take personal responsibility for your actions.

At its core, the ICP is science based, and it is deliberately formatted as a *research study*. It will soon become clear that the purpose of all research is to make causal predictions about future behaviors. The ICP methodology is designed to provide effective strategies to help you counteract the influence of outside variables (e.g., the stress in your environment that leads to emotional eating intended to temporarily soothe the stress). These variables may operate in tandem with natural and genetic predispositions toward overeating and may be playing significant roles in your inability to control your weight. Providing incremental opportunities to make comparisons with previously held beliefs and extensively rehearsed failed dieting methods is intentionally designed to facilitate a painless segue to the ICP mind-set. This strategy will permit you to remove the encumbering preexisting cobwebs more effectively.

6

♦

ALL DIETS WORK IF YOU CAN STAY ON THEM

SHARED-IN-COMMON DIETING ATTRIBUTES

There are shared characteristics and dynamics inherent within all weight-loss programs. At the onset, all diets are typically your friend and ally. The structure that starting a newly begun diet program offers is usually comforting and reassuring—a support system that empowers you to proceed. As recently as yesterday, when some emotional stress emerged in your life, you'd resort to your old, familiar habit of self-soothing through the use of comfort foods. You probably realized on some level that all these *nonhunger* eating events were causing you to feel out of control, and thus miserable, and you were most likely aware these eating habits were causing your weight gain. Yet you succumbed anyway. But today, your new diet (I'm not referring to the ICP) tells you exactly what you need to do to counteract the temptation to eat at those times that have nothing whatsoever to do with being hungry.

Every weight-loss system involves highly regulated decision-making parameters. The moment your diet begins, adherence to *food rules* is the starting point for implementing a range of associated self-regulatory tactics for controlling your weight. This is a regimentation built into whatever diet you're on; it makes all your decisions for you. Thinking is not involved, and the mindless regimentation is comforting.

All weight-loss plans incorporate *self-correcting* features for dealing with times when random events cause us to deviate from our goals. Using body weight as a reference point has always been the most effective indicator that control over one's maladaptive eating behaviors has or has not been achieved.

In the early 1940s, the British Royal Navy developed a ground-based radio navigational system for use during the Second World War. This original design transformed into what it's called today: the global positioning system (GPS). Currently, this system is used to compute an exact location from a receiver using navigational equations, and changes in location can be tracked. Functioning in much the same way as a GPS, food rules indicate the most advantageous route to your weight-loss destination, and the scale acts as a moving tracking mechanism that measures the effects of your food choices and shows whether or not you're on course.

Attention to body weight by using the scale as a measurement tool tends to promote more rational eating behaviors while increasing the probability of complying with the food rules required by whatever program you're following. Your personalized GPS uses body weight as the means to make you most aware of the cause-and-effect implications of your eating propensities.

The scale rewards you for all your effort, so much so that you're more prone to jettison reliance upon eating as a coping mechanism. The rewards of seeing the scale go down are so strong that the immediate gratification that you've always linked with consuming foods is preempted. You become convinced that the new diet will allow you to permanently rid yourself of the self-defeating, noncompliant-type behaviors that previously provided a forever-at-the-ready comforting function in your life. Easily accessible, this handy measurement tool resides on virtually every bathroom floor. In an ideal world it functions as your personal cheering section and sustains your motivation and enthusiasm. Or at least that's the way it's supposed to work.

THE SCIENCE OF DIETING

How is it possible that the dieting industry rakes in over six hundred billion dollars annually but yields less than a 5 percent weight-loss success rate over the long term? People lose weight on a diet by following the rules but are unable to stay on the diet indefinitely. They regain the lost weight—often regaining more than they initially lost—and then try another diet. This is the *focal dieting paradox* inherent in practically every commercially mass-marketed diet program. It's like playing with a yo-yo that eventually always swings up and that you can't get to stay down. This yo-yo dieting syndrome comes from the belief that a team of presumed experts have discovered a method that will help you meet the challenges required for weight-loss success—the unspoken belief that the new dieting program being offered is the result of legitimate investigation and vetting. All the proof that's apparently needed to accredit this belief is anecdotal evidence that generally everyone on the particular program is losing weight (as opposed to bona fide scientific empirical evidence that they are losing weight and keeping it off), so obviously this new weight-loss method can be touted as the "new and revolutionary dieting breakthrough."

Ironically, this conclusion isn't far-fetched. Diets and science both have the same basic goals: researching current events and making it possible to make predictions about the future. Every weight-loss method to date (including the ICP) has the earmarks of meeting scientific expectation: adherence to rules will provide confidence that you'll be able to predict weight-loss success in your future. You will lose weight on any of the mass-marketed diets as long as you follow the rules. The fundamental defect in major dieting programs is that they only provide rules and prepackaged foods that you have to purchase and eat ad infinitum; they don't teach you how to change your eating behaviors so that you can adapt to real-world situations.

One key differentiating factor that distinguishes diets from the Immaculate Consumption Program is the research-based methodology of the ICP. When conducting any research study, predictability requires minimally three criteria: identifying or detecting a problem, developing strategies to manage it, and including a phase to resolve the problem under investigation. Any research study that fails to meet these minimal guidelines will not be deemed valid within the scientific community. Validity is determined if the research has strong predictive powers.

In order to meet the minimal criteria for what's considered a valid experimental design model, a research study must include four phases:

1. Make an observation or collect baseline data.

2. Propose a hypothesis.

3. Design and perform an experiment to test the hypothesis.

4. Analyze your data to determine whether to accept or reject the hypothesis.

MAKING AN OBSERVATION OR BASELINE DATA COLLECTION

Experts agree that the first phase of any research study must include *baseline data collection.* This stage involves gathering information before the actual experiment, or in your case, before the treatment/weight-loss phase begins.

The jumping-off or observation stage of a scientific study guides the direction one's research takes. There must be an indisputable way to determine whether current events are predictive of future events. If a wrong technique is used, it will be impossible to determine that a correct solution to your problem has been discovered. The most accurate and efficient method for researching data is to employ a mathematical system for measuring outcome data. This is the only means to determine that a correct solution to your problem has been discovered. Numbers are the only way to make sure the solution you've come up with wasn't achieved by accident. There must be a verifiable and mathematically replicable or provable means that will support the direction your research is taking.

Starting body weight, as measured by the scale, is the reference point for comparison before the treatment or weight-loss phase is introduced. Body weight afterward becomes the determining factor regarding whether the program is working or not. This number is highly visible. Highly visible data is verifiable.

PROPOSING A HYPOTHESIS:

"The formulation of the problem is often more essential that its solution."

—Albert Einstein

The starting point for the scientific inquiry of every research study takes the form of a hypothesis (i.e., an assumption). The hypothesis is a tentative explanation for a phenomenon, and it is used as a basis for further investigation. It enables the researcher to assess whether predicted behavior outcomes assumed to be true are in fact true, and its ultimate purpose is to demonstrate how to derive benefit from the research study.

A hypothesis is framed as a declarative statement that indicates the direction of one's research. Because the hypothesis sets the stage for every facet of an experiment, how it's worded is critically important. *A well-stated hypothesis eliminates vagueness so that it can be rigorously tested.* The initial hypothesis for your weight-loss experiment may be stated thusly: adherence to the ICP treatment protocol will result in weight loss during the first month. Outcome data must provide complete confidence that weight-loss changes are attributable to the treatment and nothing else. Numbers from your bathroom scale will provide you with empirical proof to determine whether the hypothesis is confirmed or not.

DESIGNING AND PERFORMING AN EXPERIMENT TO TEST THE HYPOTHESIS

After proposing a hypothesis, the next stage of the research study is to design and perform an experiment to test the hypothesis. This begins the treatment phase, which, for your experiment, is the weight-loss phase. From this point forward, you'll be continually assessing whether the proposed solution to your problem (i.e., the ICP treatment protocol) is effective. Using the scale to measure body weight is an essential element in this phase of your research.

The ICP methodology helps you identify variables predictive of a successful weight-loss outcome by researching a solution to losing weight as stated in the initial hypothesis. For the purpose of your particular experiment, the design includes a way to assess whether comparison of the baseline data and the outcome data (i.e., body weight) confirms the initial hypothesis—that is, whether adherence to the treatment protocol resulted in weight loss. Comparison of body weight after the treatment makes it possible to assess the strengths and limitations of behaviors consistent and inconsistent with your weight-loss goal. The specific techniques provided by the ICP, discussed in later chapters, will help you confirm the direction to take for accomplishing your weight-loss goal.

ANALYZING YOUR DATA TO DETERMINE WHETHER TO ACCEPT OR REJECT THE HYPOTHESIS:

All research studies include a trial-and-error phase. Testing and retesting the hypothesis will be an ongoing process. This process, which will subsequently be clearly and systematically explained and modeled, helps you assess whether the observable outcome data confirms the initial hypothesis—that is, whether adherence to the ICP protocol resulted in weight loss during the first month of treatment. Having an opportunity to endure and delay goal achievement–type thoughts and behaviors begins during the hypothesis-testing stage of your research. Using information derived from direct observation, you'll be able to analyze the strengths and limitations of behaviors consistent and inconsistent with your weight-loss goals. Data from the scale is necessary to determine whether you're meeting your goals. The primary purpose of hypothesis testing is to ensure you are able to make accurate causal predictions from personal data gathered during the treatment phase.

THE SINGLE-SUBJECT RESEARCH DESIGN

At this juncture, the template used in ICP parallels every other weight-loss method. As is the case with other programs, the ICP acknowledges that the scale is the most accurate, effective, and convenient way to measure the effect of weight loss–type behaviors and to predict the outcome of your weight-loss experiment. Body-weight data is a key component in the data you'll be collecting and is used for the purpose of correlating and being attentive to behaviors consistent with the scientific study that you'll be conducting. Every modern-day weight-loss method ever offered relies on the scale as a cue for reinforcing the self-regulatory strategies for weight control. There's no way to get around it: initial body weight is the baseline number and serves as the "en route" or mediating measurement that shows whether you're moving toward your goal.

Here's the problem: what began as a tool for objective measurement of outcome has evolved into the symbolic representation of dieting success or failure. In other words, the scale has become an external reinforcement. Using the scale as the one and only way to measure outcome has become the downfall for virtually every dieter. Yes, the scale is an effective measurement tool, but its shortcoming is its external reinforcement qualities, and this characteristic makes reliance upon the scale a double-edged sword.

Due to high visibility, external reinforcements are the most powerful ways to generate behavioral changes, but unfortunately, their effects are very short-lived. The first time the scale fails to meet your expectations, there is no external reinforcement strong enough to help you manage your disappointment about a missed expectation. External reinforcements will not work in the long run as they do not provide an ongoing effective strategy for regaining a sense of equilibrium that allows you to recover, get back on track, and reorient toward your goal. Reliance on external reinforcements eviscerates one's capacity to take true responsibility for one's own actions.

Unlike external reinforcements, developing internal reinforcement strategies promotes introspective-type cognitions (or insights) that have been shown to help manage resistance when changes in your modus operandi are required. All the research to date has proven that people who are able to evaluate their own problematic eating situations and develop strategies and tactics to effectively handle those situations are more likely to maintain weight loss. Any program that fails to help you transition from external to internal reinforcement strategies at the point of consumption (i.e., the moment you eat something) is doomed from the start.

For a program to be effective, you must be able to outweigh the influence of outside variables (e.g., environmental stressors leading to emotional eating and the natural predispositions to overeat). Learning and implementing an internal reinforcement strategy will give you the insight to recognize that the scale's lower numbers represent the tangible positive effects of a successful program, nothing more (for example, taking four deep breaths will enable you to feel that your body and mind are in control of your eating behavior). Initially, however, you must reconcile being dependent on the scale as a measurement tool—while keeping in mind its limitations and vagaries. The scale is an external reinforcement as opposed to your ultimately acquiring an internal measurement of success, which will take time for you to develop.

This brings into focus your ability to evaluate the long-term outcome. Taking responsibility for your actions and developing self-management skills for permanent habit formations can and must be learned. The most applicable research design that will enable you to accomplish this is the *single-subject method of data collection* advocated in the Immaculate Consumption Program. This type of scientific inquiry has been shown to be the most effectual means for attaining self-understanding, insight, and efficient, goal-directed eating behaviors.

The first step is making the distinction between the underlying patterns of your dieting belief system and replacing them with research-based tactics that will enable you to identify your individual needs. This distinction will be guided by your experiences and derived from self-recorded observations. Self-recorded data has been shown to be the most efficacious means for attaining self-understanding. This begins your individualized method for losing weight that is at the core of the ICP.

The ICP methodology allows you to identify your particular counterproductive eating behaviors and strategically replace them with more productive ones by utilizing a specialized data collection system based on the aforementioned *single-subject research design*. This methodology brings objectivity to your weight-loss–related beliefs and behaviors and provides a strategy to accurately identify what changes need to be made and how to make them. The ICP's single-subject research design thus becomes the launching pad for taking responsibility for your relationship with food on a moment-to-moment basis.

This research methodology is what radically differentiates the ICP from every other weight-loss method. Most often, the first unplanned eating event initiates an unrecoverable relapse from the externally imposed food rules of a diet. Not so with the ICP. The ICP factors in the eventuality of unplanned eating events, which provides you with a procedure to recover from a regression (i.e., any deviation from what you consider goal achievement–type behavior). Ultimately, the ICP system will enable you to discard external reinforcement strategies and develop internal reinforcement strategies (i.e., an internal locus of control) for lifelong weight management.

As stated, the ICP follows a single-subject or individualized research design. The only accepted model for such a research design is the "A-B" collection of data. Baseline data collection is the "A" phase of your experiment, which is conducted before the treatment phase begins. The "B" phase is the treatment. The classic single-subject research design has three attributes:

1. The data collection is derived from your own observations and your own experiences.

2. By implementing a research study, you'll arrive at self-discoveries, thus making it possible to identify and alter eating habits that are more aligned and attuned with your goals.

3. Compliance with a personalized research study provides an internal locus of control rather than an external locus of control (i.e., being told what to do).

The data-gathering approach uses a *continuous assessment exercise*; that is, behaviors will be observed repeatedly over the course of the treatment. This will ensure that the treatment effects are observed for a long enough period of time to convince the researcher (you) that the treatment is producing a lasting, positive effect.

The single-subject research design involves focusing on the variability in data. Because behavior is assessed repeatedly, this design allows you to see how consistently the treatment changes your behavior from day to day. The goals of the data collection method are to:

• Identify predictors of effective treatment outcome so it's possible to tailor a program based on individual needs; and

• Develop a personal weight-loss profile that offers the opportunity to research which behaviors are consistent and inconsistent with goal achievement.

The fundamental purpose of scientific inquiry is to accurately predict future outcome—imperative when dealing with weight management. The ICP provides a research-based methodology for accurately assessing whether your eating habits and behaviors are consistent with your weight-loss and weight-management goals. The way to meet the challenges associated with developing the behaviors required for immediate and long-term weight-loss success hinges on the degree to which you make your eating behaviors discernible. The ICP provides a methodology to help you do just that.

7

◆

VISIBLE INFORMATION
IS IDENTIFIABLE

You can't continue to eat the way you are now if you want to lose weight. If you want to lose weight and keep it off, it's really quite easy. All you need to do is eat when hungry and stop when sated. Unfortunately, food's anesthetizing qualities make this highly unlikely. Typically, those who are overweight deal with stress by eating. The scientific community views this cause and effect eating phenomenon as a *paired association.* In other words, you feel better when you eat in reaction to stressful events. Because food is generally readily accessible, this makes it one of the most frequently used methods to self-soothe.

The fact is that self-soothing with food works. But it's a double-edged sword because using food for self-soothing is a leading cause of overconsumption. "Experts" in the dieting field consider this dynamic to be insidious and directly associate the phenomenon with precipitating the downfall of virtually every diet. If food in the mouth feels good, and science has proved its effectiveness as a palliative, how is it possible for you to stop using it to feel better when you're stressed? The fact is, you don't have to! If it works, why shouldn't it be used to make you feel better? Any weight-management method that fails to ask this key question is doomed.

The Immaculate Consumption Program considers self-soothing with food to be a normal coping strategy. All you need to do is ask thin people if they eat when they are not hungry as a way to feel better. If they are forth-right, they will assuredly answer "Yes!" If permanent weight management is your goal, coping with stress-related eating must be your number-one consideration. The key is not to turn away from self-soothing food behaviors but to decrease the frequency with which you exhibit them. The ICP provides a method for supporting and managing ways to self-soothe with food while at the same time helping you stay on track with your weight-loss and weight-management goals.

Having to cope with food permeates every area of our daily lives. The ICP methodology for gathering data makes this dynamic visible and allows you to access personal information about all your food-related behaviors. The systematic data-collection exercise of the ICP encourages self-awareness by exposing your dieting behaviors. Self-reflection and a heightening of your sense of consciousness and conscientiousness are the requisites for developing self-control skills. It's important to recognize whether you're predisposed to pig out on Reese's Peanut Butter Cups when you're watching *Law and Order Special Victims Unit* and whether you want to develop a strategy to manage this behavior.

Unlike a diet, the ICP accepts the fact that food in the mouth is one of the most powerful ways to cope with discomfort. Confidence with your own self-management skills will provide an internal reinforcement schedule (more about this later) that will eventually become more powerful than the immediate gratification of food. This will in turn become the impetus for eventually researching and modifying current eating behaviors while implementing the ICP.

LEARNING FROM YOUR OWN EXPERIENCES

The ICP's specialized data-collection system is designed to help you navigate through a self-recorded journey of personal discovery. This methodology prepares you for learning how to use information gathered from personal experiences in order to promote behavioral changes regarding eating events. Self-reporting makes personal information visible, which is a prerequisite to developing the ability to learn from your own experiences. And the mere act of self-reporting engenders greater feelings of self-control, which enhances motivation and enthusiasm.

Observations make current weight loss–related beliefs and behaviors visible. Instead of following orders based on the precepts of a prescribed diet, you must learn how to be guided by your experiences derived from observations that are verifiable and, therefore, provable. Another name for this procedure is incorporating "scientific law." Self-reporting is the only way to identify with accuracy what changes you need to make and how to make them. This becomes the springboard for taking responsibility for your relationship with food on a moment-to-moment basis. The ultimate goal is to help you learn from personal eating experiences and by so doing segue from an external reward system (based upon what the scale says) to an internal reward system.

MASTERING SELF-EXAMINATION SKILLS

Weight-loss sustainability is the Achilles heel of every diet. The erratic nature of life creates a 100 percent probability that a random and unplanned eating event will occur in your future. These events are often justified by the thought: "I've been doing so well that one bite of any taboo food won't hurt." Yet over 95 percent of the time, unplanned eating events begin a relapse into old patterns of eating. The result could become what's called an *unrecoverable relapse*.

This failure results from the fact that no weight-loss method other than the ICP teaches the consumer how to incorporate and integrate skills to manage potentially hazardous *high-risk events* (i.e., behaviors associated with dieting failures, such as unplanned eating). The mismanagement of high-risk behaviors is the looming downfall of all other weight-loss programs.

The ICP takes off where all other weight-loss programs have failed. Its hallmark is to provide you with the capacity to endure, adapt, and recover from each and every impromptu and unintended negative eating episode you are likely to encounter. Whenever a setback occurs, you'll know exactly what to do to get back on track. Learning effective recovery tactics requires that you develop specialized skills to assume personal accountability at the moment of consumption.

Individuals capable of viewing current behaviors are more likely to be successful when a lapse occurs. Taking corrective actions to get back on course is the result of utilizing self-observation skills. Self-observation is likely to make the lapse temporary, rather than trigger an unrecoverable relapse.

Your eating behaviors are made more visible through a detailed data-gathering system. Preconceived notions are acknowledged, goals are determined, and expectations are realized. The ICP provides an ongoing and systematic navigation protocol through and around memories that reflect your past dieting experiences.

The ability to objectively access normal and everyday eating patterns provides a detailed roadmap for accessing current food-related behaviors, and it serves as a guide for determining what's required to attain future weight-loss goals. Viewing spontaneous occurrences objectively and using the information already at hand is the only way to survey and navigate experiences and make the kinds of judicious decisions necessary for the ongoing management of food-related events.

Recording information accurately encourages insight, paving the way for a sense of self-control—the requisite upon which the ICP is based. The result will be enhanced management behaviors at the moment of consumption.

Remember, at present it's unrealistic to think you'll be capable of reversing your embedded dieting belief system. Challenging these beliefs at the outset will only create doubt, fear, and resistance to any incoming information. The result is likely to be noncompliant-type thoughts and behaviors. This must be prevented at all costs. The ICP's Intake Stage (i.e., the baseline data-gathering phase) discussed in the next chapter is specifically designed to avoid challenging previously held beliefs at this juncture

A SCIENTIFIC MODEL FOR BEHAVIORAL CHANGE

In the mid-nineteenth century, William James wrote a scientific article describing how to develop good habits and break bad ones. Today, many consider his paper to be the first scientific application for how to deal with problems associated with human behaviors. He wrote, "Success at the outset is imperative. Failure is apt to dampen the energy of all future attempts, whereas past successes nerve one to future vigor." Consistent with James's theory, the ICP attempts to make sure weight-loss success is realized from the start.

The scientific model for behavioral change must describe concepts in a way to ensure that you, the research subject, have a clear understanding of how current and future food-related behaviors will be addressed, analyzed, and managed.

The ICP protocol begins with a baseline data-gathering stage (the Intake Stage). This stage involves collection of personal data by answering a series of innocuous-type questions. Although the questions might not seem worthy of any special attention, don't be fooled. What might appear to be unremarkable answers to innocuous questions will supply the data necessary to research solutions to problems under investigation. When done correctly, information obtained through the Intake Stage is the foundation for learning how to replicate solutions to food-related issues by systematically referring back to the hypothesis and determining whether adherence with the ICP is helping you realize your weight-loss goal.

As a properly designed experiment, outcome data (body weight) will provide complete confidence that weight loss is attributable to the treatment and nothing else. The hypothesis will then be accepted as a provable fact. Provable facts are imperative as a way to limit the intrusion of erroneous or ineffective conclusions.

After all the baseline data has been accumulated and the hypothesis has been stated, the treatment phase begins. Through a continuous/ongoing assessment exercise, behaviors will be observed over and over again as a way to determine if each and every food-related decision is consistent or inconsistent with goal achievement–type actions. Data from the Intake Stage is used for comparison to assure that the treatment effects are observed for a long enough period of time to convince you that adherence with the ICP has led to success.

8

◆

DATA GATHERING FOR
PERSONALIZED RESEARCH

The following section comprises the baseline data–gathering phase that, in the clinical setting, is the Intake Stage. The Immaculate Consumption Program begins with a scientifically controlled inquiry stage as a way to research solutions to the problem under investigation. This phase is *not* the treatment (or weight-loss) phase that will be introduced subsequently, and it is *not* performed for the purpose of understanding or drawing conclusions about current eating behaviors. Rather, this phase involves an Intake Exercise that documents baseline data—body weight, dieting history, and eating patterns—before any treatment is introduced.

The ICP adheres to the scientific-experimental model. Following the baseline data–gathering protocol of a scientific study enables the researcher (you) to observe behaviors under investigation objectively in order to test the hypothesis for the research being conducted. Objective observation of current behaviors serves as the standard of comparison from which all future progress will be judged. Consistent with a *scientifically controlled inquiry protocol*, the function of the Intake Exercise is to state and clarify personal information. There is no interpretation of the data at this point. However, this data-gathering phase does help prepare you to accurately document personal and individualized experiences, which will be useful during the treatment phase.

This Intake Stage is basically a systematic record-keeping exercise that includes:

- Retrieval of historic dieting memories while attending to current thoughts, feelings, and behaviors.

- Self-recording personal information, which makes past and current behaviors more visible.

The Intake Exercise is derived from a well-defined assessment protocol that will make your dieting belief system discernible by chronicling readily accessible personal information. This protocol is simply a recipe based on the following guidelines:

- Information collected before the treatment begins (e.g., body weight) will be compared with similar information collected during and after the treatment (the ICP) is introduced.

- Baseline data determines criteria for evaluating the program's outcome objective.

The following Intake Data Sheet provides all data necessary during the treatment phase and will allow you to strategically research whether the hypothesis is realized or not. Upon completion of this Intake Stage, the data will be the basis of comparison for all your future research.

THE INTAKE EXERCISE: COMPLETING THE INTAKE DATA SHEET

The following Intake Exercise provides the Intake Data Sheet, which is an experience-based retrieval system. (You may want to use a spiral notebook to record your responses and not try to write your more lengthy answers in this book to the subsequently more complex questions that appear later. You may also choose to record your data on your computer or tablet.) Keep in mind that each answer to the following questions will help you view personal data systematically and more objectively. Whenever you see this symbol (*) pay extra attention—you're about to be provided with a rationale for researching and testing your hypothesis, and you will also be provided with a scientific explanation designed to positively influence your current dieting belief system.

STEP #1: GENDER / AGE / HEIGHT

Male/Female: _____; Age: _____ Height: _____

STEP #2: ESTIMATED WEIGHT

Write down estimated weight _____

Estimating weight before actually getting on the scale is an exercise in hypothesis testing. The hypothesis or assumption before getting on the scale will then be proven or disproven when you actually weigh yourself. This scientifically accepted research protocol will support greater objectivity while your personal weight-loss profile is evolving. Keep in mind that the hypothesis is a tentative answer to your weight-loss problem. Applying the treatment plan over and over again is the only way to demonstrate its effectiveness. These issues will be extensively addressed and clarified in the next chapter.

STEP #3: USING THE SCALE

The only way to find a solution to the challenges of losing weight and maintaining weight loss is by defining the problem specifically enough so you can determine whether you are going in the right direction. After completing the Intake Stage, an appropriate hypothesis will be crafted that will enable you to determine—indisputably—the direction your research is taking based on outcome data (body weight) provided by the scale.

At this point, and throughout the following month, the scale will be the tool that determines the direction you're heading. This reliance on the scale as the exclusive measuring mechanism allows you to strengthen your association with losing weight. For one month, assessing body weight will be the single criterion for assessing whether you've met your weight-loss expectations.

IT'S TIME TO GET ON THE SCALE

Write down current body weight: _____

At this juncture, body weight is merely the comparison reference point to determine the direction you're going. The scale will be the measurable indicator that reveals how past weight-loss experiences have influenced your current expectations for what's required to lose weight. By bringing your belief patterns to the surface, the scale provides a guide for incrementally modifying what you have previously taken for granted—a necessity to attain your weight-loss goals.

STEP #4: WEIGHT-LOSS EXPECTATIONS

    a.   Ideally, how much would you like to weigh? _____

    b.   What suit or dress or pants size would you then wear? _____

    c.   What size do you wear now? _____

Decades of actuarial research have enabled insurance companies to assign risk factors for diabetes, heart condition, and strokes based on a person's height and weight. This is the most economically effective way for insurance companies to determine premiums that each person should pay. The result of such actuarial research has led more and more consumers to use numbers from height-weight charts or body mass index (BMI) charts as benchmarks to determine weight-loss success or failure.

Many consumers have made the effort to adapt and meet the expectations of the medical standards regarding what's considered to be healthy based on height-weight and/or BMI charts because:

- They are convinced that they are not healthy if they don't meet the standards that height-weight charts and/or BMI charts deem to indicate normal health.

- They feel pressured into conforming to the actuarial standards stated in height-weight and/or BMI charts.

An individual's decision that he or she has met goal weight expectations is often based on data from a normal-population study (e.g., a height-weight chart or BMI chart) that fails to take into consideration individual factors. The determination of a normal population is simply that—it is a statement of a statistical norm. Any particular individual may have a healthy body weight despite deviation from the statistical norm. This is why it is imperative that you determine if data from actuarial studies are valid or unreliable markers for your personal physical and emotional health.

There are many physical, behavioral, and emotional markers that may not fit the "normal" population but work best for you. Developing a trusting relationship with a medical doctor who's supportive of your program will provide the kind of feedback that will enable you to take responsibility for what's required to have an ongoing healthy weight-loss experience.

STEP #5: PRETREATMENT GOALS

   a. How much weight would you like to try losing each week?

   _____

   b. If you lost less weight one week, how would you feel? _____

   _____

   (Explain in as much detail as possible.)

   c. How would you react if you don't meet your weekly weight-loss expectations but are losing weight consistently? _____

   _____

   (Explain in as much detail as possible.)

When asked these questions, most dieters feel a typical goal is a one-to two-pound weight loss per week and would be disappointed with less. You'll soon come to appreciate why losing weight more slowly is correlated with attaining long-term goals.

STEP #6: DIETING HISTORY

Assessing information from past dieting attempts will help determine if the behaviors are consistent or inconsistent with goal achievement (i.e., weight loss). There is no way to get around the fact that, at the first stage of any weight-loss method (including the ICP), goal achievement is determined by one thing and one thing only: eating differently than before. At this stage, you should not tamper with your current dieting belief system. As previously stated, your accustomed diet-type mind-set about losing weight is a powerful reinforcement at this juncture and should be sustained.

Learning something new not only depends on what's remembered from past dieting attempts, but also depends on information currently filtering in; therefore, the meaning of a new concept must interface with previously stored concepts. When reviewing weight-loss history, relevant facts are frequently overlooked. The inability to recall details accurately typically has no bearing on ultimate success or failure. Most often, you will recall forgotten data as you proceed with this exercise.

The habits of dieting reflect all the beliefs and opinions that each person harbors concerning what it will take to lose weight. These habits usually make it impossible to change the perception that going on a diet is the only way to accomplish weight-loss goals. Thus, we will acknowledge past weight-loss experiences during this section of the ICP Intake Exercise.

The following questions document the history of your weight-loss attempts. Their purpose is to accumulate information to determine how your particular weight-loss patterns fit together. When you finish answering these questions, you will be able to evaluate how well you have been managing problematic eating situations.

DESCRIBE YOUR FIRST WEIGHT-LOSS ATTEMPT BY PROVIDING THE FOLLOWING DETAILS

What year? _____ How old were you? _____

Name or method: _____

Supervised or not? _____

What was your starting weight? _____

What was your weight on completion? _____

How long did it take to get to that weight? _____

How long did you stay there? _____

How long did it take to regain the lost weight? _____

Now describe each of your other weight-loss attempts, in consecutive order to the most recent attempt, by answering these questions for each attempt.

In this step, you'll state only those eating behaviors that were consistent with what you believed complied with weight-loss rules that resulted in the scale going down. This information includes only your externally imposed dieting behaviors. Information gathered here will result in determining those habitual features that have come to define your unique model for losing weight. These questions are designed to make the details of your past dieting attempts highly visible. The more observable and transparent your thoughts, feelings, and behaviors are, the more you can control them. Accessing current thoughts, feelings, and behaviors more accurately is the gateway to developing more productive self-management strategies and tactics.

Your immediate goal is and has always been to lose weight. In answering these questions, you will likely discover that all these diets helped you lose weight, but you were never able to keep the weight off. The issue then becomes: if diets don't work to keep the weight off, what does? You will soon become convinced that the answer to this question is the ICP.

STEP #7 EXPECTATIONS FROM SELF AND OTHERS

This step addresses social and environmental issues revolving around your food choices.

Name anyone you might eat with regularly who is familiar with your eating habits: _____

Will this person be supportive of your goal achievement–type behaviors, and if so, how? _____

STEP #8 CURRENT EATING PATTERNS

The following questions should only include examples of what you have come to believe as diet-type eating days that are classified as "good" diet days or in-control eating days. *Good diet days* represent those times when you felt in control of all your food choices—those times when you were confident that you were going in the direction you wanted to go.

The following series of questions involves only days you experience as good diet days. There might be different types of days, such as weekdays, that might include working versus weekends and holidays. Try to give as complete a description as possible for what these days look like:

What time do you usually get out of bed in the morning? _____

Do you consume any liquid or food at this time? _____

If not, what is the time of your first meal? _____

Give an example of a good diet or in-control first meal: _____

_____

Do you have a snack before lunch? _____ Give as many examples as the types of snack or snacks eaten: _____

_____

List the time lunch occurs: _____ Give details of what you typically eat, and again, give as many examples of a "good day" lunch as possible: _____

_____

Do you have a snack before dinner? _____ At what time? _____

What does that snack consist of? Give as many examples as possible:

_____

_____

What time is dinner? _____

Give examples of a diet-type meal, including beverages and dessert:

_____

_____

Do you have a snack after dinner and before bedtime? _____

What is that snack? _____

You need to determine what behaviors indicate that you've gone off track. You must remind yourself that you're in the process of learning how to be a researcher. This means that concepts must be made visible so you can measure and quantify them to get the basic data required to begin your experiment. Factors that are objective and concrete are more easily measured. Careful and exhaustive investigation of the evidence of a definable problem will help you find a solution.

Now it's time to go back and answer every previous question, but this time only include what you consider to be "bad" or "nondiet" eating days.

Eventually you'll be able to view eating behaviors in a neutral and noncritical manner. You will realize that overeating is comprised of learned food habits that are at odds with your weight-loss goals. All it will take for successful (i.e., permanent) weight reduction is for you to examine meticulously your embedded counterproductive food-related habits and replace them with ones that are more congruent with your current goals. The ICP will show you how to accomplish this.

STEP #9: TEN PROBLEMATIC FOODS OR EATING BEHAVIORS

You need to take many factors into consideration for the successful management of your weight. The questions posed for this step and the next step are in preparation for the start of the ICP treatment phase. Their purpose is to help you devise effective ways to research your current eating patterns and develop a *minimal intervention strategy* to adequately meet your nutritional needs while working toward your weight-loss goals.

Name ten foods or situations that cause you to feel bad about your eating behavior: _____

_____

_____

_____

_____

_____

_____

Include food, beverages, and any behavior that you perceive as counterproductive to what you're trying to accomplish. The way to determine your answers is to ask yourself: "When I exhibit this behavior, does it make me feel bad and/or out of control?" or "Will eating this prevent me from reaching my goal?"

STEP #10: REASONS FOR LOSING WEIGHT

Give as many reasons as possible why you want to lose weight:

_____

_____

_____

_____

_____

_____

_____

_____

_____

_____

_____

From all your reasons, indicate the number-one reason why you'd like to lose weight: _____

_____

_____

Now that you have completed the Intake Exercise, and it's time to begin the experiment (i.e., the treatment phase). In the following chapters, you'll be shown how to apply two scientifically proven learning behaviors that are the foundation of the ICP. The result: you'll be able to redirect dependencies on external motivators to a comprehensive holistic approach that will ultimately become your *Personalized Internal Reward System.* By so doing, you will learn to develop an internal locus of control. All the information from this point onward will be used to create internal reinforcement schedules linked to the outcome data that the scale provides.

9

♦

BEGINNING
THE TREATMENT PROGRAM

REVISITING DEIDRE

When we last left Deidre, I was in the process of asking her a series of questions about her modus operandi. These questions were an integral part of the intake process. I was about to ask her the one last question that would complete the personal data-gathering phase of her intake.

This question involves going over the ten-item list from intake question number nine (Ten Problematic Foods or Eating Behaviors). From the ten-item list, name one high-calorie food you eat frequently that causes you to feel bad or upset. The dynamic might present as follows:

- After taking the first bite of this one food you can't stop.

- The mere thought of eating this food produces anxiety.

- It requires extreme willpower, self-control, and goal-directed motivation to resist the temptation to eat this food item.

- Not eating the food causes you to feel deprived, perhaps even depressed.

- Eating this food causes you to feel out of control.

- You realize you may never safely eat this one food item when dieting.

- If and when you eat this food, it feels as if the weight-loss phase has been a failure.

- The mere fact of craving this food item suggests that an unrecoverable relapse may have begun.

The first principle the ICP addresses is how craving responses occur and how to manage them—permanently. Through classical conditioning, Pavlov got a dog to salivate in response to a bell. Prior to this research, salivation had been considered reflexive or automatic, a response that cannot be controlled. Originally, the bell was a neutral stimulus, meaning that it hadn't caused any reaction whatsoever from the animal. When pairing the bell with some meat powder, however, the dog salivated 100 percent of the time. By the end of the experiment, the dog would salivate upon hearing the bell before any meat powder was provided. Thus, the dog exhibited a salivary response to the bell, which the dog had previously experienced as a neutral stimulus.

How does this apply to overeating? Classical conditioning guidelines enabled researchers to determine that the eating behavior of overweight individuals is not typically dictated so much by hunger, but rather by environmental or external cues. This implies a lack of awareness of, an insensitivity to, and/or a disregard of internal physiological cues.

Behavioral techniques have become the universally accepted way to control the embedded phenomenon revealed in Pavlov's groundbreaking research. Consonant with what had now become a scientifically accepted theory, therapists treating obese patients sought behavioral interventions as a way to help them manage overeating episodes.

In the late 1960s, Dr. R. B. Stuart initiated an early behavioral weight-loss intervention. He sparked academic interest by seeking to modify fundamental health-related counterproductive eating behaviors internalized by his clients. In the field of obesity treatment, behavioral interventions were now thought to be especially effective in bringing about weight reduction. Weight Watchers designed its weight-loss program based on Stuart's 1967 research on behavioral self-control procedures for overeating. Investigations beginning in the 1970s by Dr. Albert Stunkard and others began questioning the long-term efficacy of behavioral treatment programs for obesity.

Unlike other behavioral treatment programs (such as Weight Watchers, Nutrisystem, etc.) that rely on a multifaceted treatment procedure incorporating far-reaching lifestyle changes, the ICP extinguishes nonadherence by researching only one obstacle that has interfered with weight reduction and weight maintenance.

The following question to Deidre addresses the first rule of the ICP and completes the personal data-gathering phase of her intake:

Me: Of the ten problematic foods you identified, which one are you willing to give up? It shouldn't be your favorite food. The food you want to consider is the one food that, when you take the first bite, you can't stop.

Deidre: I was told about the "contract" food and have been thinking about it. I know it should be bakery goods. The thing is, they're my favorites, and I don't know if it's possible for me to *not* eat them.

Me: The contract-food rule is the result of proven scientific outcomes based on classical conditioning and deconditioning principles. So before answering, it's important that you have a basic understanding of how Pavlov's research applies to permanent weight-loss sustainability. Based on Pavlov's research, when a food is given up, the desire or craving for that item begins to diminish. The "extinguish craving graph" below shows that the longer you don't eat something, the more the craving for it diminishes.

You'll notice that once you stop eating something, the salivation or, in more human terms, the craving is extinguished. Extinction takes about three weeks. The key is to stop eating it completely, because eating it just once will restimulate the craving for that food. One paired association is all it takes for a salivation response to be reinitiated.

If you commit to 100 percent compliance to your self-determined, voluntary behavioral change (i.e., giving up one highly problematic food), you can accomplish something that no other weight-loss method has ever provided. You will learn how to recover from what you've always considered poor food-choice decisions that you've believed to be antithetical to attaining your long-term weight-loss and weight-management goals. Until now, the downfall of every other weight-reduction program you've tried has been the inability to recover from what you've always identified as a course-changing dieting misstep, otherwise termed an unrecoverable regression. The ICP methodology offers a science-based solution to this dreaded, and all too common, self-sabotaging phenomenon.

Take a look at the following graph. You eat something that you crave. Since you've had bakery goods recently, it's impossible *not* to salivate at the thought of eating them. Believe me, within the first day, without a doubt the craving for whatever item is given up begins to diminish. Notice on the graph that it's not at equal intervals. The third week shows a dramatic drop in the craving response.

PAVLOV'S EXTINCTION GRAPH:
CRAVING—EXTINCTION CURVE

- *100% Salivary and craving response for contract food*
  - *First Week not eating it – Thinking about food evokes a salivary response for it*
    - *Second Week – Salivary response lowered but desire/craving still alive*
      - *Third Week – Desire/craving gone but sight still—mmm !*
        - *Third Month – Sight doesn't evoke desire/craving Smelling might still evoke salivation*
          - *One Year – Desire/craving and salivation for contract food extinguished*

Me: Deidre, close your eyes. Now imagine your favorite bakery item is right in front of you. What's that like?

Deidre: Mmm! I can taste it.

Me: Virtually every diet derived from the medical model of disease views overeating as a disruption in or deviation from biological norms, and they attribute this phenomenon to a physical or chemical cause. The result is the embedded belief that overconsumption is a food addiction that has to be cured. Addictions to heroin, cocaine, or alcohol are managed in one way: the drug of choice must be completely and permanently given up. Because it is impossible to give up food, dieters have been forced to manage overeating-type behaviors with willpower and self-control, thus insuring that for all intents and purposes, the capacity to resist temptations will ultimately reach its breaking point over the long run. Dieters relying on self-control exclusively are setting themselves up for all but inevitable failure, because willpower can only be stretched so far.

I give my word that you'll lose the desire for whatever you give up. When you give up the food entirely, you'll no longer respond to the craving for that food. The stimulus-response cycle will be broken, and the craving will fade away. If you exhibit 100 percent compliance (especially during the first month) from this point onward, my guarantee is that at no time will you ever have to rely on willpower or self-control. If, however, you do not exhibit 100 percent compliance, there will be a perpetual craving for that food item.

Deidre: It's my favorite food, and I'm afraid a time will come when I'll succumb to it. I know myself. I would feel like such a failure, and I would be so ashamed that I wouldn't be able to face you ever again. I'm setting myself up to fail even before getting started.

Me: Is there a bakery good that you have a particular problem with?

Deidre: Anything containing chocolate.

Me: Are you saying that if a bakery item doesn't include chocolate, it's not a problem?

Deidre: Yes, definitely. Without chocolate, I'm really not very interested in it.

Me: What about chocolate as your contract item? You can have candy, ice cream, and bakery items as long as they don't contain chocolate. That way you're not giving up all your favorite foods.

Deidre: That sounds terrific and too easy, except for one thing. It will break my mother's heart if she can't buy me a chocolate cake for my birthday, and I'm not willing to do that.

Me: When is your birthday?

Deidre: November 13th.

Me: Today is June 8th. Your birthday is six months from now. So you're willing to give up everything chocolate except on your birthday?

Deidre: I can definitely do that.

Me: It's time for me to take out a piece of paper and write a very simple and specific food contract:

I will not eat anything chocolate, including candy, ice cream, and bakery goods, with the exception of cake on my birthday, November 13th.

Signature: _____ *Date:* _____

Deidre: So you're telling me if I want to lose weight and keep it off for the rest of my life, all I need to do is write my food down before I eat? And other than chocolate, I can eat whatever I want?

Me: Yes.

Deidre: This is too easy. I don't see any possible way this can ever work.* But I know it has for others, and I will sign and date my contract.

---

*People who make a comment like this have the highest success rate. They've complied with both rules of the ICP, suggesting not only are they feeling no resistance toward the program, the effortlessness in some ways suggests they're not doing enough and, hence, are willing to do a lot more.

10

◆

CURRENT BEHAVIORS SERVE AS OBJECTS OF INVESTIGATION

Permanent habit formations can be created by developing the ability to learn from personal experiences as opposed to being told what to do. The most effective way to accomplish this is following the bottom-up approach. This approach gives people the opportunity to assume responsibility for their own learning process by meticulously exploring their personal actions, and in so doing, provide the means for true changes to occur.

Each person must be encouraged to research, acquire information, and pursue a direction needed to achieve his or her goal. Researching personal actions rather than relying on following food rules dictated by others, creates learning experiences that comprise the foundation for the development of self-organization skills. This is the only way to develop permanent behavioral changes.

You are about to learn and apply a scientific experimentation method that will, in due course, enable you to access your current behaviors and thoughts in order to implement a scientific research study designed to allow you to make accurate and precise predictions about future events. This chapter brings you to the heart of the ICP method and furnishes guidelines for proceeding with personalized research in a scientific experiment. It will ultimately put you on the path to creating your own individualized weight-loss and weight-management plan.

OBSERVING AND INVESTIGATING
PERSONAL FOOD-RELATED BEHAVIORS

Behavior therapy offers many techniques to assist with personal growth. Often, behavior therapists deal with behaviors considered maladaptive; that is, behaviors that are self-defeating and/or interfere in some way with the welfare of others. Outcome data from various scientific and empirical research studies shows that controlled behavioral therapy is often successful in helping people establish self-monitoring techniques and improve their lives.

This type of therapy assumes counterproductive behaviors are learned and, therefore, can be unlearned through a series of techniques. Making maladaptive patterns perceptible can lead to initiating lifestyle changes and help people learn how to manage and control their self-defeating behaviors. The emergence, application, and viability of behavioral therapy explains why it became in the early 20th century the leading modality for dealing with the obese population.

There is a ledger-keeping system in the ICP, but first you must be taught a way of precisely documenting your eating behaviors that will have positive long-term effectiveness. The ICP provides a unique modus operandi for tying psychological phenomena to objective physical food-related events. Chapter 13 will show how to integrate this information into the comprehensive internally based measurement process upon which the ICP is based. Deirdre's actual ledger will be used to demonstrate the actual application of both ICP rules (giving up one food and ledger keeping).

It is accurate to say that high visibility of all food-related decisions is the only gateway to develop the skills required to predict and ultimately manage unplanned eating events. Accessible information becomes the reference point for evaluating how your past weight-loss experiences have contributed to your current expectations for what's required to lose weight. If you want the scale to go down, you must eat less than you're eating now. All that's required is finding an eating plan that offers fewer calories than you're consuming currently, and in all likelihood, the scale will reward you. The first month is about this "scale rewarding" stage of weight loss. What makes the ICP different than any other ledger-keeping weight-loss method ever offered will soon become evident.

RETURNING TO DEIDRE

I tell Deidre that, from this point onward, the second part of the ICP will make up 95 percent of her weight reduction phase. There has to be an identification method that makes current eating behaviors visible. Visibility de-randomizes the intrusive perturbations (emotional noise) that can push you off course and interfere with goal achievement.

> *Me*: I'm going to teach you a method of observation that will equip you to detect and investigate your personal food-related behaviors. My role is not to analyze the information you provide but, rather, to facilitate the investigative and analytical process. I'm about to show you the ledger—an assessment tool for making all food-related behaviors visible. Accessing patterns and beliefs will make it possible for you to become an objective observer of all your food-related attitudes and behaviors. Ledger keeping based on behavior-modification principles begins your systematic journey of self-exploration.
>
> "From wherever the mind wanders due to its flickering and unsteady nature, one must certainly withdraw it and bring it back under control of self."   *—Bahagavad Gita*

FOOD CONSUMPTION LEDGER

Overeating is based on three proven facts:

1. Motivation to overeat is instinctual (i.e., it is an involuntary reflex).
2. Eating for self-soothing works as a coping strategy.
3. There's a 100 percent probability that random and unplanned eating events will occur.

If the motivation to overeat is involuntary and eating to self-soothe works, plus there's a 100 percent probability that random and unplanned eating will occur, how is weight-loss sustainability possible? The medical/disease model views overeating as being reflexive. Reflexes have always been considered automatic, indicating there's no time to think about what we're about to do. This suggests we have no control over our biological need to self-soothe by eating—a premise addressed extensively in the following section.

The ICP views overconsumption as a *learned response* for coping with stressors. If something can be learned, it's also possible to unlearn it. The ledger you're about to begin relies on a cognitive/behavioral protocol for studying habits more consistent with what you're trying to accomplish— namely, to unlearn some current behaviors that have prevented you from a successful weight-loss experience.

The number-one indicator for permanent habit formations is the ability to adhere to the offered treatment protocols. The problem is that treatment rules are often based on the *if-then* protocol: *if* you follow the eating plan, *then* you'll succeed with your weight-loss goals. As mentioned earlier, so-called dieting experts have erroneously concluded that the only way to realize weight loss is by strict compliance with sanctioned, well-established food rules.

The National Weight Control Registry (NWCR) serves as the bedrock for the if-then approach to weight loss. As discussed in Chapter 4, analysis of the registry data detected five major behaviors of people with long-term weight-loss maintenance. As mentioned earlier, these have been coined "convincing indicators." The conclusion resulting from the NWCR data analysis was that *if* you adhere to these five behaviors, *then* you can also join the ranks of successful weight maintainers. Research indicates that adherence to treatment rules is positively correlated with meeting weight-loss expectations. Here's the rub: unfortunately, what all the research fails to show is that meeting other people's expectations makes adherence and compliance unlikely.

Right from the start of the ICP, you will be compelled to think about each of your food choices. Permanent habit formations will only occur by developing the capacity to access an experience-based retrieval system; that is, the ability to rely on firsthand observations and experiences. This is what the ledger is designed to accomplish. Your experiences will be accessible for the purposes of future reference, comparison, and guidance. Nonadaptive and counterproductive thoughts, feelings, and behaviors must be replaced with new ones that are more attuned with attaining your weight-loss goal. This will only occur when you develop your ability to retrieve the relevant data from your ledger and apply it productively to current experiences and counterproductive eating behavior.

The ledger's systematic data-collection process encourages self-awareness through making dieting behaviors visible. Self-reflection provides a level of conscientiousness—the foundation for self-control skills. And self-control is the foundational principle upon which the ICP is based. Confidence with self-management skills at the moment of consumption becomes a kind of reinforcement schedule more powerful than the immediate gratification of food. This makes the ICP what it is.

The ICP is not a diet but, rather, a training manual for permanent habit formation. First, perceptions of eating behaviors are made more discernible. Through detailed data gathering, preconceived notions are acknowledged, expectations are realized, and goals will be determined and stated. The ledger provides a systematic navigation procedure through and around memories regarding your historic dieting experiences.

The ledger is based on a well-defined assessment protocol that will make your dieting belief system evident by enabling you to readily access personal information. Learning new ways of eating is made possible by viewing and researching personal food-related behaviors so that you can increase the frequency of your taking complete responsibility for your actions before, during, and after the moment of consumption.

By the end of the first month, you'll be consciously evaluating all your eating behaviors. You will need to buy a notebook that you will carry with you at all times. Your ledger will provide a detailed record of all foods eaten. The date goes along the top of the page for each day. Entries include the eating time, eating activity/location, food eaten, and the size of the portion, the calories in that portion, and a rating of the degree of hunger and preference for that food on a five-point scale. The following details the experienced-based retrieval system (i.e., the ledger) that will make you confident that you can influence and control every eating event.

DATE

Time	Activity/Location	Food/Portion	Calories	Hunger*	Preference*

*Hunger and Preference rating numbers are detailed below.

DATE

- Date is entered once each day. The day begins when you wake up (after-midnight foods are included with the previous day).

TIME

- Record time eating begins.

ACTIVITY / LOCATION

- If you eat the item alone in the kitchen, write "alone in kitchen." If you are in a restaurant, record the name of the restaurant. In most other cases, there will be some activity to record (e.g., watching TV, reading, talking on the phone with family, having lunch at work, etc.).

FOOD / PORTION

- Include the description of each food item and estimate the size of the portion in ounces, cups, tablespoons, etc.

CALORIES

- Estimate the calories for each food item.

At this point, try to estimate calories as best you can. If you've never paid attention to calories before, purchase a food scale and a comprehensive calorie-listing manual to get an accurate assessment of the calorie content in your food. The good news is that the ability to visually estimate food quantities with relative accuracy happens very quickly. Weighing an item one or two times is really all that's needed. Estimating as closely as you can the foods and liquids that you consume is important, but what's even more important is consistency in the recording procedure.

The validity of the caloric management of food has been clearly established for decades. If calorie intake is lowered, then the scale will go down. Measuring calories has become the most accepted and well-recognized system for losing weight. The fact is, if you want to lose weight, you must eat less than you're eating at your current weight. The one and only basic way to lose weight is through the caloric management of your food intake.

As indicated above, the ICP has a calorie-counting component, but it's not actually a calorie-counting program! Caloric assessment is only one element in a more holistic and comprehensive behavior-modification methodology; it serves as a functional tool for achieving your weight-loss goal and works in tandem with other distinctive ICP techniques. Here, you don't have to comply with a certain caloric ceiling; instead, calories are used as a research device to determine how to best get your needs met. Assessing calorie consumption begins your experimental study: investigating how to combine the goal of losing weight with the goal of maintaining your weight loss. Calories will be relied on as a convenient measurement instrument so that you can create a personalized model for losing and sustaining your weight.

HUNGER

You will be assessing your current state of hunger on a five-point scale:

0—I can easily not eat.

1—I can easily wait a few hours to eat.

2—I can easily wait one hour to eat.

3—I need to eat now; if I wait any longer, I'll be too hungry.

4—I've waited to eat one hour too long.

5—I've waited to eat a few hours too long.

Do the best you can at this juncture. The fact of the matter is that most people have no idea what hunger really feels like. During the first three weeks, through a systematic analysis of Deidre's ledger in Chapter 13, you'll slowly begin to be able to differentiate between hunger and appetite. True hunger is a *need* to eat. Appetite is a *desire* to eat. You can be at a zero level of hunger but still have an appetite or desire to eat. Trust that, at this point in the ledger-keeping procedure, you will be reassessing all your numbers during the next few weeks. It's a fact that the more weight you need to lose, the longer it will take to correctly calibrate your assessment of hunger.

PEOPLE WHO HAVE FIVE TO TEN POUNDS TO LOSE

- Could take anywhere from one to three months to begin to correct their assessment of hunger.

PEOPLE WHO HAVE TEN TO TWENTY POUNDS TO LOSE

- Could take anywhere from one to eight or nine months to begin to feel confident with assigning a hunger number.

PEOPLE WHO HAVE TWENTY OR MORE POUNDS TO LOSE

- Could take between three months to a year to accurately assess hunger.

There are a variety of reasons why we eat besides hunger. An actual feeling of hunger is very, very fleeting and almost ghost-like. One moment you might feel as if you're starving, and a second later the feeling is gone. The ICP is designed to ultimately help you determine your true hunger level. The preference number, which will be discussed next, will be of use concomitantly in allowing you to assess this level more precisely. Chapter 13 will show how to correctly distinguish between hunger and appetite.

The goal of ledger keeping is to make nonthinking eating patterns highly detectible. The preference column of your ledger begins what's called a "successive approximation to the goal" exercise. Successful compliance with the ICP rests on your ability to go from unthinking eating behaviors to conscientious ones. The only effective way to assure adherence from the onset is to provide a method to easily assess a food-related thought. Once you can experience the evaluation procedure prior to the moment of consumption as being natural and unobtrusive, success is practically guaranteed.

Awareness of a pivotal food choice must proceed through a quick analytical process that is practically unnoticeable and instantaneous. For this reason, the preference column includes the simplest and most unobtrusive means for stating a food fact. Assigning a preference number is nothing more than an exercise for determining how food is categorized in what is called the lowest level of data abstraction.

The hunger and preference columns will provide data to eventually determine the difference between actual biological hunger ("I need to eat") and appetite ("I have a desire to eat").

PREFERENCE

The following five-point scale indicates how much you like or crave one food over another:

0—The least preferable food. I'd have to be at a "five" hunger to consider eating this item. If I'm invited to my boss's house, and this food item is served, I'd make an excuse not to eat it.

1—Very slight preference, but I would never order it at a restaurant, and if I were offered a taste, I would decline.

2—I would prefer it over a food with a "one" preference rating but could easily substitute another item for it. If a friend offered me a taste, I would be willing to try it, but that would be the extent of ever eating this food.

3—This is a likeable food, but I could easily substitute another item for it.

4—There are times when I might crave this food. If and when I do have a desire for it, substituting something else would take some effort.

5—I crave this food item. When I want it, nothing else will do.

The most important thing about the preference number is that once you assign a number to the food item, it becomes that item's permanent number. This is very, very important. For the first three weeks, the preference number is actually the most important number—again, since it's most easily accessible.

Keeping the preference number permanent acts as an *object constant* and becomes the reference point for making the distinction between hunger and appetite. "Object constant" describes the tendency for objects to be perceived as unchanging despite variations in the positions and conditions under which they're perceived. How the principle of object constant determines the distinction between hunger and appetite will be discussed in Chapter 13, through the systematic analysis of Deidre's personal ledger.

During the first month, the preference number acts as a measurement indicative of a craving or appetite response. Toward the end of the first month, it will become evident that high cravings or a high desire for a specific item might not have anything whatsoever to do with being hungry.

The ICP will require that you keep a ledger, but you will be shown the correct way to document eating behaviors when using it. First, you aren't expected to keep a food diary to comply with eating rules someone else dictates. Second, *how* the ledger is used differentiates this ICP ledger program from all others.

I tell Deidre that the ledger is an "operant conditioning" or "pre-entering before eating" procedure. This means that you cannot eat anything until your ledger is completely filled out. Based on the principle of contingency management, any eating behavior for the first month of treatment becomes *contingent* upon writing down in your food ledger *beforehand*. Writing food down before eating is a declaration of what you intend to do. Writing down afterward is merely confessing a behavior you've already done. The principle of contingency management is described extensively in Chapter 13 as we systematically evaluate Deidre's ledger.

Those who show 100 percent compliance for one month with both requirements of the ICP—not eating one food item (i.e., the contract food) and writing food down before eating (i.e., completing the ledger)—have the highest success in the first month of treatment. Making a written record *before* eating will eliminate the possibility of automatic or nonthinking food-related behaviors. Those who exhibit 100 percent compliance with both rules also showed the highest probability for long-term weight loss and weight maintenance.

Monday's appointment is over, and Deidre leaves my office after agreeing to adhere to both requirements of the ICP. Our next appointment is on Wednesday. That next meeting, discussed in the following chapter, will begin the systematic application of the ICP.

11

◆

THE INITIAL TREATMENT SESSION

REFLECTIONS AFTER MONDAY INTAKE SESSION

Deidre leaves my office, and I begin recording my notes for the Monday intake session. From the first phone contact until completing the intake session, for all the reasons previously discussed, I'm confident that Deidre is the real deal and is a terrific candidate for the Immaculate Consumption Program. After completing my clinical notes, I close Deidre's folder and begin planning Wednesday's session.

While it's my conjecture that Deidre will do just fine, there's always the possibility she won't. All the work we've both done so far is no guarantee that Deidre will have what it takes to make permanent changes in her food-related behaviors. This requires that she research and ultimately transform certain ways of thinking and acting with regard to her food choices, creating new eating habits that are more consistent with her weight-loss and weight-maintenance goals. The bottom line is that without effective self-management skills, it's not possible for her to be prepared and equipped to deal with problem situations that are guaranteed to occur in her future.

Wednesday's appointment will help both of us evaluate whether she will benefit from what I'm offering her. For now, 100 percent compliance with both behaviors required by the ICP (i.e., giving up one item and ledger keeping) is the most accurate predictor for weight-loss success. It's always important to consider that desperation, which is typical at the onset of any program, would seemingly assure the dieter's compliance with the rules. Since Deidre fits the profile, I'm confident she'll lose weight this first month. But I'm still concerned about her long-term success. She has many bridges to cross.

Because the ICP is unlike anything Deidre's ever undertaken before, it can be somewhat unnerving. As opposed to familiar dieting rules, now her success requires adhering to a program that involves learning and applying two proven scientific principles for making behavioral changes. Since she won't be following a regimented eating plan, the first few sessions can be anxiety producing, because she doesn't know yet how the program actually works.

The most common client experiences prior to the next appointment are feelings of vulnerability combined with a lack of confidence. I'm counting on the fact Deidre's come to believe this is the only game in town for a successful weight-loss event. Clients are generally in a state of hyper responsiveness when beginning the ICP, thus making it more likely for them to accept new and unique types of information and dynamics.

Feelings of dependency on me in my role as mentor and guide are unavoidable during the first few weeks of treatment. But if I've done my job properly, Deidre will show up for Wednesday's appointment ready to see me as a compassionate taskmaster capable of leading her in the direction she needs to go. Early-onset dependency is not only unavoidable, but it's also a necessary component when beginning any weight-loss method. On the other hand, long-term dependency can be problematic.

For this reason, maintaining a student-teacher role for too long is counterproductive. It inhibits clients from learning how to incorporate self-management techniques and from taking responsibility for their own eating behaviors. Accordingly, the ICP is strategically designed to make sure that the taskmaster (i.e., therapist) begins to incrementally surrender her hold during the first month of the program.

When it comes to learning a new habit, there's one universally agreed-upon fact: if something feels good, we are likely to repeat it. In all likelihood, we will not repeat an experience or behavior that feels bad. Consequently, during the subsequent meticulous analysis of Deidre's ledger, it's imperative that her first self-exploration experience be a positive one. After Wednesday's session, Deidre will have a greater appreciation and understanding of the role that the contract food and her ledger play in making this happen.

My job is to help Deidre research behaviors to determine which are consistent and inconsistent with her goals. Turning to measurable data is the most effective way to accomplish this. Each and every behavior will become a way to target actions that move her from a theoretical to an experiential conceptualization about how the ICP will benefit her.

WEDNESDAY APPOINTMENT—THE INITIAL TREATMENT SESSION

I open the front door and am greatly relieved when Deidre shows up for our Wednesday appointment on the dot. It's an indicator of her likely success in the ICP. While it may appear insignificant, punctuality is a strong signal that someone is willing to take responsibility for his or her personal actions. My taskmaster role will become obsolete at some point, thus enabling Deidre to make the ICP her own and perceive it as not being mine or anyone else's.

As usual, the three of us (with my dog leading the way) walk toward my office. I point out to Deidre that her punctuality is a sign of respect for me and for her commitment to the ICP. I also tell her that this is actually a behavioral marker that my doctoral research substantiated as signifying the strong potential for future sustained weight-loss success.

But the significance of being on time has always been a no-brainer for Deidre. What has been a normal and regular responsible behavior for her on a daily basis has now been brought to her attention and acknowledged. This makes her feel proud and fosters a realization that there are other positive attributes within her that need to be identified, recognized, and reinforced.

I am about to ask Deidre to get on the scale. At the onset of any weight-loss method, the scale's descending numbers act as the primary motivator for the client to change his or her current ways of eating, and as mentioned previously, make noncompliance with the two rules unlikely. Noncompliance from the start would be the equivalent of striking out in the first inning.

As far as Deidre's concerned, the numbers registered on the scale verify that she's done exactly what she was supposed to do. Deidre is about to reveal the success or possible failure of the initial phase of her weight-loss program. Being sensitive to her likely performance anxiety, I purposefully make the request as nonchalantly as possible: "Before we sit down, why don't you step on the scale?"

Based on previous observations, I assume that Deidra has followed the program with 100 percent compliance since our last session on Monday. I wasn't surprised when the scale showed a loss of three and one-quarter pounds. While this seems like a lot, this kind of loss is consistent with clients who were in the process of gaining weight right before starting the program. Since most foods are sodium bearing, just a little reduction in these foods produces significant losses at first. If this kind of loss goes beyond the first week or two, it indicates that clients are putting themselves on self-imposed supplemental diets, which in the final analysis will prove counterproductive. This will become evident very quickly. Clients who show no weight loss or gain at this point can be another matter.

As an aside, several years earlier a client named Monica came in for a consultation. She explained that, although her best friend Ann had been raving about the program for months, she had still been reluctant to make an appointment. Overweight all her life, Monica was never able to stay on any diet longer than two weeks. After watching Ann keep off more than twenty-five pounds for over a year, Monica wanted to give it one more try.

Monica proved to be a highly vigilant client. She weighed, measured, and wrote down all foods beforehand. And though she had eaten no contract food, she showed up for that first Wednesday's appointment with no weight loss. By the end of the second week, there was still no loss. Although she was discouraged, her friend's demonstrable success somehow enabled her to give ICP "one more week."

In the third week, Monica came in and, lo and behold, the scale went down three-quarters of a pound. It wasn't much, but it was still something. It turned out that Monica showed a weight loss between one-half and three-quarters of a pound every three weeks. It didn't matter what she did, the scale stayed stuck until the third week. Most would have given up with such minimal success. Other programs she tried didn't factor in Monica's weight-loss pattern, and she had often been accused of fibbing about what she was actually eating. But she was absolutely thrilled at her every-three-week weight loss. It wasn't much of a win, though it was consistent and predictable. Monica now had the exact equation for losing weight.

Still, success at the beginning is imperative. The scale going down is a key motivational element during the first few weeks. It's proof that the ICP is working and proof of Deidre's success in using the program. The ICP is designed so that initial weight loss is all but guaranteed for anyone who has adhered to the program, even after only a day and a half.

Just as important, this accomplishment is verification that Deidre has complied with the rules. While the immediate reinforcement of her weight loss is important, it's also imperative to begin the process of incrementally de-emphasizing the scale component. Deidre has now proven to herself that she's capable of losing weight, and it's true that early success is correlated with future success. At this point in time, however, there is no way to restrain the flawed inclination to link the *loss of body weight* with *sustainable weight loss.*

Deidre must begin the process of breaking her emotional ties with the scale and her dependency on it. It's important to find a way to distract her from her excitement about losing weight and divert it to another goal-achievement mind-set. This is why, while she was still standing on the scale, I asked her: "Are you getting enough food to eat?"

This forces Deidre to consider her answer to my question, and by so doing, immediately shifts her attention away from the scale. It requires her to initiate an introspective modality and to decide if she is indeed consuming enough food. Determining whether her needs are being met becomes a stimulus for her to pay attention to her current eating patterns. By asking her to consider her situation from a more holistic point of view—that is, if she is getting her eating needs met—I am strategically steering Deidre to use her recorded personal data as an alternative means for assessing the efficacy of the program, rather than having her rely exclusively on the scale.

Deidre responds, "Yeah. I'm getting enough food to eat. I was really hungry last night—actually both nights after dinner. This is my hungry time. It's actually a combination of my hungry time and my bored time, and I am aware of this. I try to have things to do at night to keep busy. But the fact is, in comparison to all my other diets, it actually felt like I overate."

I reiterate to Deidre that 100 percent adherence to the ICP method practically makes it impossible for her *not* to lose weight.

At all times, it's important to remember that one of the first month's key objectives is to help de-emotionalize the scale. The very first issue I address with Deidre after the weigh-in is the importance of assessing the numbers on the scale with greater objectivity. I tell her it's not possible to determine the actual cause of weight loss after only one-and-a-half days. Eventually, she'll learn how to use data from the scale effectively, but during the first few weeks this is unlikely.

> *Me*: To lose a pound of body fat means you have to burn thirty-five hundred calories. You're down three pounds, meaning you would have had to burn 10,500 calories over what you require for your daily maintenance. It's not possible to get an accurate picture at this point, since most of your loss includes water-weight loss.

> *Deidre*: How many calories should I be eating?

> *Me*: That's impossible to know at this point. During the first several weeks, your job is to research caloric consumption that contributes to weight loss, weight gain, and weight maintenance. In the first month of treatment, 60 to 70 percent of loss is based on water weight. So, it's impossible at this stage to make a distinction between the loss of water versus adipose (i.e., fat) weight.

There is no way to determine the cause for your weight loss at this moment. Again, since 99 percent of food contains sodium, water retention or loss isn't a conclusive measurement of achieving long-term weight-loss goals. Just changing some food choices often cuts out a lot of the salt people consume. Eventually, we need to have the data necessary to research what will contribute to losing, maintaining, and gaining weight, but we're really not addressing caloric ceilings now. Rest assured that after several weeks we'll have that information available.

Whatever you're doing appears to be working, but still, the number-one focus of your research has to be ways that will ensure you're getting your hunger needs met. During the next several weeks, you'll also figure out the caloric range to meet your weight-loss goal.

I sit down in my leather recliner, while my dog makes himself comfy in his bed under my desk. I tell Deidre to get comfortable, and she kicks off her shoes so she can rest her feet on the couch. My next question is the same question I pose to every client: "Did you eat your contract food?"

My clients are unaware that I make it a practice not to deposit their check for one month. If a client replies to my question, "Well, it was someone's birthday at work, and I didn't want to hurt her feelings, so I had just a tiny bite," I would flag that response and put aside that person's check. I'd see her for maybe a week or two to confirm my suspicions, but at some point if my suspicions are confirmed, I would tell her as gently as possible that she isn't ready to begin the program and return the check.

Nonadherence with the contract-food agreement is the number-one indicator that someone is not a good candidate for the ICP. Mind you, I've never actually told a client that he or she is not a good candidate. Instead, I diplomatically say, "It's not the right time to start."

As I suspected, Deidre says she didn't eat her contract food. I then ask her what that was like for her.

> *Deidre*: A coworker down the hall from me has a big glass jar of Hershey's Kisses. I made a point not to walk past her desk. I stayed away from the break room, since there's always chocolate candy in there. Also, at dinner last night while watching TV, a commercial for chocolate came on. I jumped up and ran into the other room. I just didn't want to see it.

> *Me*: Why is all that significant?

> *Deidre*: I'm serious about the contract we made. I just didn't want to see any chocolate. I wouldn't break my word, but I knew seeing it would make me nervous.

> *Me*: Did you feel deprived by having to rely on willpower at any time?

> *Deidre*: Huh. Now that I'm thinking about it, there was no willpower involved. I made a contract with you, and I wasn't going to break it. It was something else, but I really don't know what it was.

It would be normal for Deidre or anyone going through the program to feel initially as if she were merely following orders, but she would soon begin to appreciate that when you stop eating something, you stop craving it. Not eating one food provides a sense of being able to control a craving that only last week was unmanageable. It takes only a day or two for the process of salivary extinction or cessation (i.e., a craving response) for that food to begin to take hold. Within a few weeks, it is indisputable that cravings for that particular food will be demonstrably diminished.

The previous week, just thinking about the contract food would have elicited Deidre's craving for it. Going to bed the first night after not eating it proves that it's possible to quickly achieve one behavioral change in the food-consumption modus operandi. The subsequent sense of accomplishment is the result of exerting control over one food that only yesterday was problematic. Immediately, a sense of well-being results from adhering to the contract. The craving is replaced with the reinforcing effects experienced as an indisputable sense of achievement. *The need for willpower or self-control strategies to control the craving for Deidre's contract food are no longer required.*

It will become apparent how giving up one item creates feelings of control that become the foundation for making behavioral changes. This induces an inner reinforcement so powerful that the immediate gratification the particular food item heretofore furnished loses its power over us permanently.

Since Deidre didn't eat any chocolate foods, I proceed to determine how her ledger keeping is progressing. Deidre has only completed her ledger for one-and-a-half days, but still, I pose the following question:

Me: Overall, if 100 percent is perfect, with no empty columns, what's your percentage of recording in your ledger before you eat?

Based on all behaviors she's exhibited so far, as I expected, Deidre responds: "100 percent." I then pose a multipart question soliciting her overall perception of the ICP.

Me: Overall, how would you describe the program so far, such as: "I think it's good or bad, I love or hate it, I feel different or no different?"

Deidre: I love it. I've written down my food with other diets but never before eating. That's why this is not like anything I've ever done before. I woke up this morning feeling excited, but, to be completely honest, I also felt very anxious. I'm not sure if I'm doing it right.

Me: I'd be surprised if you weren't confused. Since all you've ever experienced is traditional dieting, it is impossible for you not to compare what you've done since Monday with your past experiences.

Prior to going over all the personal information contained in Deidre's ledger, it's important that she become an informed participant, so she's prepared for what to expect. My discussion regarding the program follows a specific protocol. First, I inform Deidre about not eating her contract food. Next, I tell her that there should be no empty spaces in her ledger, which would indicate she's not following the protocol. Since the primary focus of attention for the first month is to improve the technical integrity of Deidre's ledger, most of the data from her ledger will be continually revised.

Now I remind Deidre that the focus of her attention should be the process of keeping her ledger rather than robotically following a plethora of dictated food rules. The OCD (obsessive compulsive disorder)-type focus on my part, combined with all the data she's providing, makes it possible for us to be on the same page and know exactly what we're each bringing to the table.

I point out to Deidre that this will be the first time we'll be going over personal eating behaviors. I also tell her that by the end of this session she'll have a greater appreciation that her ledger is merely a feedback system to interpret information she's providing. I give her my word that she'll leave the session with greater confidence about how the program works.

Even before opening her ledger, I convey to Deidre how I used to unwittingly trigger negative reactions from my clients when going over the information. It seemed obvious to me that my clients' defensiveness was because they were ashamed of their eating behaviors. What appeared to be resistance was occurring too frequently, and it caused me to consider whether I was a contributing factor for such obvious discomfort. Were my questions and how I was asking them unintentionally causing anxiety?

Then it dawned on me: at the onset of every weight-loss attempt, dieters are desperate, thus making it likely they'll be compliant and follow the rules. For the first few weeks, Deidre could be expected to go to great lengths to make sure she's meeting expectations. This is what I'm counting on. Desperation is an effective motivator for reducing the probability of deviating from any behavior seen as consistent with weight-loss goals. At the same time, anything that might have the earmarks of criticism is off-putting to those always in the habit of meeting others' expectations. I clearly need to alert Deidre about what will follow in order to avoid triggering excessive anxiety, which would be counterproductive and cause phobic reactions to our analysis of her ledger.

Me: We're about to nitpick every entry. Much of the recorded information today is likely to be changed.

Before I even begin going over the entries, I point out to Deidre that what appears to be critical questioning of her data is not nitpicking. Rather, it reflects my commitment to making sure we're both on the same page in understanding and assessing the information recorded in her ledger. What appears to be an obsessive-type questioning process is my desire to fully comprehend exactly what she's trying to convey.

In thinking back about my own past dieting failures, I recalled a situation when my mentor in graduate school was going over my personal eating patterns for the first time, and I vividly remembered that it had triggered powerful negative emotions. I realized that past dieting failures contribute to feelings of embarrassment and shame. It's normal that there's a hypersensitivity to anything that smacks of criticism about food choices. This personal experience makes me especially empathic about the way in which I handle this critically important interaction with clients. Been there, done that.

Managing feelings of defensiveness is imperative at this point, and I inform Deidre it's imperative that I know exactly what's going on in her mind so I can address her issues and concerns.

After I explain the rationale for my seemingly hypercritical approach, no one has ever reported being harshly censured or denigrated. Rather than feeling belittled, people trust that my job is to help them think more clearly about their eating behaviors. Deidre is being prepared to more objectively question, analyze, and modify the information she has recorded in her ledger.

12

◆

HISTORICAL ANTECEDENTS
OF MODERN-DAY DIETING

Keys in hand, Deidre was about to unlock the front door to her mother's house. This happened over four years ago, when she was still dieting. She was joining her family for dinner and was confident that the infamous Pink Box would be sitting on the kitchen counter. Normally, she wouldn't give a second thought to having a few cookies or a piece of cake, but tonight was different. Having followed her latest diet scrupulously for three weeks, Deidre had lost seven pounds. Any serious dieter would be reluctant to do anything that might compromise this indisputable success, especially during the first few weeks of a new diet.

Deidre realized there would be instances in the future when she might not follow the diet's rules precisely, but she thought that wouldn't pose a problem for a long time. She would rely on willpower and self-control, which made her confident she'd able to overcome any predisposition to overindulge that particular evening.

Current behaviors provide the basis for what eventually becomes historical data. The ability to trace the lineage of what makes up current weight-loss beliefs and behaviors will contribute to putting your current weight-loss expectations into historical perspective. Adherence-type rules and associated behaviors owe their origins to dieting precepts that were initiated more than a century ago.

DETECTION OF THE OBESITY PROBLEM

In the early nineteen hundreds, insurance companies began to notice higher payouts for medical claims and earlier-than-anticipated payouts for death benefits. Actuarial or statistical descriptions were used to determine the likelihood of possible health risks in an insured's future. For insurance companies, calculating risks required a highly specialized formula, utilizing the *if-then* equation, so that policyholders received a fair return on respective insurance investments while, at the same time, not causing financial ruin for insurers. A specific way to measure and categorize individuals was required in order to identify them and assign them to certain risk categories. *If* people fit a particular medical profile, *then* it was possible to predict higher medical costs would be incurred.

The more accurate the data-collection phase, the more reliable the outcome data would be. And the more accurate the data, the greater confidence insurers could have in determining premiums that represented precise predictions about future health risks for the insured. Parenthetically, the *if-then* studies for insurance premiums became the foundation for how data collection and analysis should proceed in scientific communities. These correlation-type methods of data collection and analysis set the standard for what constituted a worthy scientific experiment. Data had to be collected and measured based on precise measurements. Only then could science realize the goal of insurance companies: accurate prediction of future events.

There had to be a better measuring device to more accurately collect and analyze data and determine the factors responsible for the economic losses in the life- and health-insurance industry. The more definable and measurable the data, the more precise the correlation could be made about precipitating factors. It was fiscally imperative that insurance companies devise a means to more accurately identify and measure the underlying causal data.

The universal standard for weight measurement was established in Europe in 1837. The following year, in Great Britain, Richard Salter patented the spring scale. Today's doctors' scale, with that familiar series of marks at regular intervals, is based on that early technology.

This numerical ranking of body weight is the single factor most closely associated with dieting. In effect, the scale *detected* the problem of being overweight. It was now necessary to come up with a way of determining the statistical calculation that would allow insurance companies to assign the insured into risk categories.

The medical establishment and the insurance industry considered the scale to be a precise and scientific means for applying objective classification standards. It provided a method of measurement that enabled insurance companies to devise a mediating or "en route" system to determine the statistical calculation of risks. The mediating system was called the Heights and Weights Chart. This standard measurement assessment tool profiled and categorized people in an attempt to predict health risks. *If* people fit within a certain height and weight range, *then* it was possible to statistically determine their future health risks. Premiums were established based on what was considered to be indisputable evidence.

The correlation of outcome data revealed to insurance companies that cardiovascular disease and many other health-related illnesses were also on the rise. Further actuarial studies proved that obesity was the culprit and resulted in the earlier payout of death benefits. As a result, obesity was rated the fastest-growing health problem in this country and the greatest source of a wide range of health-related conditions. Further outcome data predicted that *if* obesity weren't cured, *then* there would be the potential for devastating economic consequences in the United States. The scale became a reliable identification tool for successfully correlating body height and weight with health risks. Actuaries had succeeded in defining a population of individuals with the potential financial risks insurance companies might incur. Obesity was on the rise. As predicted, it was slowly becoming an epidemic.

Scientists revisited the work of the eighteenth-century French scientist Antoine Lavoisier. In 1780, using a guinea pig to measure heat production as a way to measure energy (or calories) in food, Lavoisier devised a mathematical formula that could be easily calculated. Measuring energy (or calories), he came up with the name "calorimeter" for a device to determine how many calories are consumed when eating. All diets follow what has become this universally accepted equation: lower your calories, and you'll lose weight. This formula sets the standard for every weight-loss model.

Science's goal of predicting the future requires that a theory be explained as simply as possible. Based on this premise, in the case of weight loss, the more succinct and uncomplicated the theory is, the easier it would be for consumers to adhere to a weight-loss protocol. A mathematically formalized theory easily calculated would be ideal from the point of view of impact and functionality. Armed with statistics, physicians started advising their patients to keep their weight under control. There had to be a way to solve what was fast becoming an obesity epidemic.

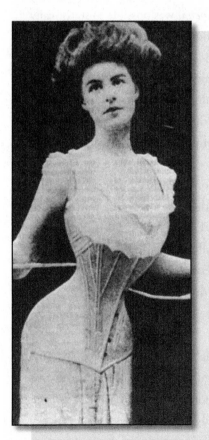

DR. LULU HUNT PETERS

The Queen of Calories and the First "Weight-Loss Guru"[1]

◆ ◆ ◆

In the early 1920s, an American doctor came up with the simple formula that brought the only voice of reason to the world of desperate dieters. Based on a precise and scientifically proven equation, there is one and only one way to lose weight: lower calories, and the scale will go down. This became the universally accepted method for weight reduction and is the only way to lose weight.

---

1   Parts of the following discussion are from Wikipedia and fall under the fair-use doctrine of United States copyright law.

Dr. Lulu Hunt Peters was a medical doctor and author who became what was considered the most well-known female physician in America of her time. A longtime overweight woman who topped out at 220 pounds but managed to lose seventy of those pounds, she was on a weight-reduction mission. Dr. Peters created a dieting method and mentality that would endure until the present day. There have been many different names and different theories for how best to implement her basic proprietary principles, but the fact is that every diet to date follows her universally accepted equation.

Based on Lavoisier's calorie-burning theory, Dr. Peters used this formula to address her personal weight problem and started advising her patients to keep their weight under control. She began seeing human bodies as "Fireless Cookers," burning energy using a specific formula that would determine what each patient was required to do to lose weight. She explained the concept of the calorie as a scientific unit of measurement of the energy potentially available from food (Gruber, Beth, *The History of Diets and Dieting Part V: The First Low Calorie Plan*).

Dr. Peters became the very first weight-loss guru by popularizing the concept of counting calories as a method of weight loss. She also wrote the first modern diet book, originally published in 1918, *Your Stomach Must Be Disciplined: Lulu Hunt Peters and the Beginnings of Calorie-Counting in Corporeal Self-Regulation, 1918–1924*. This book sold between eight hundred thousand and two million copies and was the number-four bestselling nonfiction book in 1923, according to *Publisher's Weekly*, and it was the first weight-loss book to become a bestseller (Kawash, Samira, *Candy: A Century of Panic and Pleasure* [2013]). Her book remained in the top-ten nonfiction bestselling lists from 1922 to 1926. Her calorie-counting system for losing weight is still in print and is still racking up positive reviews.

She was the first person to widely popularize the concept of counting calories as a method of weight loss (Jou, Chin, 2007 Annual Meeting of the American Studies Association). Dr. Peters became a passionate public health advocate (again, she was on a weight-loss mission) and made the dieting awareness mentality what it is today. She explains in her book that "hereafter you are going to eat calories of food. Instead of saying one slice of bread, or a piece of pie, you will say 100 calories of bread, 350 calories of pie." Women were shown how to calculate their ideal weight with a formula (Gruber, Beth). Her book included estimates of food portions that would contain one hundred calories, based on research from a variety of technical publications. This is almost the identical weight-loss method Weight Watchers relies on currently.

Dr. Peters indicated how many calories someone should eat per pound of ideal body weight (similar to the body-mass index used today). She paid less attention to the issues of what sorts of foods a person should eat. Under her system, a person of Peters' height could eat whatever she wanted, as long as she maintained a strict diet of twelve hundred calories per day. She often warned against eating candy, because she felt women who ate a little would end up bingeing on it. The concept of cutting back calories was touted as the best form of weight loss/weight watching for American women who wanted to conform to the modern twentieth-century leaner body image that was coming in vogue.

All diets begin in highly emotional states. Random eating behaviors from only one day before can now be controlled by getting on the scale, and having measurable data helps the dieter identify the behaviors that are consistent and inconsistent with goal achievement. There is no way to get around the fact that in the first stage of any weight-loss method, including the ICP, goal achievement is determined by one thing and one thing only: losing weight. As stated throughout this book, this objective in no way should be discounted. Losing weight initially is a powerful reinforcement and should be sustained.

Self-observation must be viewed as a positive experience at the onset of any weight-loss attempt, since this is the one and only component that will ensure compliance to the treatment protocol. The scale thus became the most effective way to institute realistic strategies for collecting, analyzing, and managing personalized identification data. Dr. Peters believed that it would make behaviors required to lose weight visible.

REVISITING THE SCALE

At first, the structure that starting a new diet offers is typically comforting and reassuring, yet excessive eating of high-calorie and/or high-carbohy-drate foods will invariably work at cross purposes with losing weight and thereby cause us to feel bad. In the past, we recognized that we were out of control and feeling miserable, because on some level we were aware that our eating habits were responsible for our weight gain. Today, we know exactly what we need to do to shed the pounds when on a diet. The regimentation built into the selected diet makes all our decisions for us. Thinking is not involved, and this regimentation is comforting. Motivation and incentive are enhanced, and the scale ideally serves as our very own cheering section.

The power of the scale derives from the fact that it has always denoted a precise assessment for the direction that our diet is taking. The numbers revealed in the little window are inviolate and cannot be impugned. All they can do is go up or down or remain the same. The data from the scale rep-resent the most accurate reference point for future comparisons of weight loss or weight gain and is the most effective indicator that control over one's overconsumption has been, or has not been, achieved.

It bears repeating that the scale is typically our friend and ally at the beginning phase of a diet—it's the support system that empowers us to proceed. During this phase, there will be times when some stressors emerge. Dependence upon the scale is what enables us to renounce our old, familiar habit of self-soothing through the use of comfort food. Why? The scale is a powerful reinforcement that rewards us for all our effort, so much so that we've jettisoned our reliance upon using food as a coping mechanism. The rewards are so strong that the immediate gratification we always associated with consuming high-calorie, nutritionally unsound foods no longer serves the previous comforting function in our lives.

Relinquishing that now-familiar habit of relying on the scale would be perilous, because it's been relied upon as the cue to reinstate the tried-and-true self-regulatory strategies for controlling weight gain. This is what evokes significant emotional responses and makes us aware of the cause-and-effect implications of our eating propensities. The more our body weight lowers, the more we're energized, which contributes to intense feelings of enthusiasm and attests to a job well done. During the initial stage of any weight-loss program, this will not change. That's why using the scale as the method to scrutinize eating behaviors under investigation must not be tampered with.

Exclusive reliance on the scale is imperative at first, but dependency on a long-term basis is detrimental for most dieters. Numbers on the scale should *never* be the only measurement of a weight-loss event. Dieters have been indoctrinated with the belief that following food rules and keeping to a caloric ceiling is the only way to achieve weight-loss success—but that's not the case. The following chapters will provide an investigative-type approach as a way to research other causal factors for changing eating patterns permanently. The shortcomings of total reliance on the scale will be discussed in greater depth below.

There is an intimate and dynamic interplay between motivation and losing weight. The scale serves to correct any behaviors that might prevent you from reaching your weight-loss goal. Losing weight acts to suppress any spontaneous thoughts or actions that lead away from compliance with more worthwhile weight-loss tasks. You have to eat differently if you want to lose weight, and it's unlikely you'll accomplish that on your own. Compliance with agreed-upon rules is and will always be the measuring stick for weight-loss success. Unfortunately, following other people's food rules does not provide the means for internalizing enduring habit patterns *that lead to permanent weight loss and weight-loss management.*

THE SHORTCOMINGS OF THE SCALE

The scale is an *external reinforcement* as previously noted. External reinforcements are highly visible and powerful and are capable of changing current behaviors quickly and efficiently, but they have a short shelf life.

The scale is a triggering stimuli, or device that functions as a cue to control food intake, but only for a while.

The scale has become an indisputable measurement of adherence or nonadherence to food rules.

It cannot be overstated that the numbers provided by the scale can unerringly indicate that we are losing weight. Here's the paradox: we need the scale, but if we use it exclusively as an external reinforcement, it's not usually enough to sustain us over the long haul. Without the scale to reward us, compliance would be nonexistent. Without compliance, it's unlikely that we would continue to pursue our weight-loss goal. It is axiomatic that successful dieters are those who follow orders and do exactly what they're supposed to do with no questions asked. As long as they stay within the diet's boundaries, they can expect to lose weight. It's when they begin to deviate and fall off the wagon (i.e., regress) that problems ensue.

At the onset of all weight-loss attempts, invoking the need for will-power, self-control, and procedures to manage resisting temptations will always elicit short-lived responses. This is the one glaring limitation of the scale: although it can inspire when it's headed south, it can demoralize when it's headed north. The message translates into the only way to lose weight or maintain weight loss is to adhere strictly to the dictates of the diet. For weight loss to continue and sustain, this requires ongoing motivation and willpower. Any lapse in either can prove perilous.

Here's the problem. At first, reliance on the scale controls our natural predisposition to succumb to eating for emotional reasons. The sole function of the scale becomes to influence or modify the process for changing the way we eat. Granted, seeing the number on the scale go down is a powerful external reinforcement. Waking up Monday morning ready and willing to make drastic changes to insure the scale's descent conveys a foreboding sense of desperation that in the long-run is destined to prove counterproductive.

The most significant shortcoming of relying on the scale as a way to control caloric intake occurs the very first time you don't get your expected reward from the scale. This is experienced as a missed expectation. In most cases, it triggers a downward spiral that culminates in a food choice that is adverse to weight-loss success.

In contrast to external reinforcements, the ICP's research-based methodology is designed to help you overcome problematic eating situations by developing internal reinforcement strategies at the moment of consumption. Behavioral changes are more likely to occur and be sustained if people are exposed to information in a way that allows them to research and pursue the direction they need to go. Transitioning from external reinforcements to an internal locus of control puts people in the driver's seat. This kind of learning experience makes self-management possible. As previously mentioned, all the research to date has proven that people with the capacity to evaluate how well they have handled problem situations and develop strategies and tactics to deal with those situations are more likely to maintain weight loss.

THE INCURABLE ILLNESS

Since the turn of the nineteenth century, there have been many attempts to fix the problem of overeating. Examples include magic potions, caloric ceilings, hypnosis, drugs, gastric bypass surgery, lap-bands, and research regarding how to control hunger by experimenting with severing hunger centers in the brains of rats. It is evident that the medical model remains the focal protocol for virtually every treatment for controlling weight. As stated, this model views being overweight as a disease that has to be cured.

Dr. Albert Stunkard was considered an iconic authority in obesity research. In 1959, he concluded that "to-date weight loss methods were showing a 95 percent failure rate." Up until the 1970s, no weight-loss program produced any long-term outcome data. In 1983, Dr. Kelly Brownell pointed out that if a strict definition for the formulation of a cure is adopted for obesity (such as a reduction to an ideal weight and maintenance at an ideal point for at least five years), an individual is more likely to recover from most forms of cancer than to satisfy these criteria. No weight-loss program or method has produced long-term outcome data for successful weight loss since 1970, except the ICP.

Successful weight-loss and weight-management systems haven't been available for one very simple reason: the medical model has convinced the public that being overweight is bad. Consistent with that model, current scientific evidence suggests that overconsumption is a disease that will never be cured. The July 2011 issue of *Discover* magazine contained an article entitled "The Hungry Brain," in which scientists claimed the only way to attack obesity was in combination with drugs. Currently scientists are doing research in deep brain stimulation as a way to curb eating behavior by producing an electrical charge to the hunger centers and thus revisiting the original 1903 study.

The World Health Organization is now focusing on prevention strategies for avoiding obesity in the younger population. Most of the research is going into education. Funding for the current population of obese people prioritizes controlling the symptoms of all the diseases incurred from being overweight. Managing such symptoms is considered economically sound, because a cure for being overweight is considered unobtainable.

The problem—until the advent of the ICP—was that there hadn't been any system to help those who are overweight transition from external to internal reinforcement strategies at the point of consumption. The traditional and sacrosanct guidelines externally imposed by a diet are intended to make the scale go down, but those guidelines clearly aren't working. All dieting programs fail over the long term, because they rely on external reinforcements, motivation, and willpower to handle unplanned, problematic eating situations.

The following chapter presents doorways for fine-tuning decision-making intersections before, during, and after every moment of consumption. A personal GPS guidance strategy will be continually available and at your disposal, pointing you in the direction you need to go and targeting your individualized weight-loss goals and procedures after only the first month.

13

◆

THE INITIAL TREATMENT SESSION— CONTINUED

As indicated previously, the rationale for writing down the required details in the ledger before eating is to eliminate automatic or semiautomatic eating. Evaluating both the caloric content of food and your hunger sets up a decision-making parameter (not yet discussed) that is quite different from following someone else's food rules. Ledger keeping is based on a *cognitive model* of behavioral change. Being compelled to think about food choices beforehand provides the ultimate *inner-reinforcement schedule* that is the foundation for developing the most effective self-control strategies.

An added motivational factor is that my ICP clients know they will be meticulously reviewing their food ledger during their next face-to-face session with me. The first time they actually analyze their ledger can evoke feelings of apprehension, and clients often have performance anxiety before this meeting.

THE FIRST TIME GOING OVER THE LEDGER

It's now time for me to go over Deidre's ledger with her. Feedback is communicated in a very specific way to prepare her for what she can expect. This helps manage the potential anxiety reactions often elicited when scrutinizing a client's eating behaviors. Initially, writing down food before eating is demanding and feels artificial. Since it is more difficult to recall information from a day or two before, we always start by reviewing recent entries first. This provides easier access and reduces performance anxiety significantly.

As you may recall, prior to looking at her ledger, I asked Deidre whether she completed 100 percent of the entries (no empty columns), and she replied that she had.

> *Deidre*: I did make some changes, and I have a lot of questions. I didn't eat my contract food, and I wrote everything down before eating. But to tell the truth, I really don't have any idea of how this works, so I don't know if I did it right.

> *Me*: We'll be changing a lot of your entries as we go over your ledger. By the end of our session, you'll feel a lot more confident about how to go forward. You told me everything was written down beforehand. Is that accurate?

> *Deidre*: Yes.

REVIEWING DEIDRE'S LEDGER

TUESDAY, APRIL 18

Time	Activity/Location	Food/Portion	Calories	Hunger*	Preference*
7:18*	Home in kitchen	Wheatena	~~175~~ 150	3	3

* This OCD-type focus surely comes across as nitpicking. But what might seem insignificant to Deidre represents detailed attention to the time entry and sets the meticulous standard for how we're about to proceed with the systematic analysis of every entry from this point onward. First, recording with precision beforehand exemplifies an immediate reinforcement for achieving journal entering precision. Second, as far as Deidre is concerned, the exactness used in the time column provides irrefutable proof she's complied with her program.

TIME COLUMN

Me: You wrote 7:18. How did you come up with that time?

Deidre: From my cell phone, because I wanted it to be as accurate as possible.

ACTIVITY/LOCATION COLUMN

Me: I see you were in the kitchen.

Deidre: When I'm home, this is the place I normally eat 90 percent of my meals.

CALORIES COLUMN

Me: You changed the calories from 175 to 150. Why?

Deidre: I measured one-third of a cup of the cereal and one-fourth cup of nonfat milk. Both came to 175 calories. After the cereal was made, it looked like too much, so I took some out and threw it away.

PREFERENCE COLUMN

Me: I see that for your Wheatena entry you wrote down a "three" preference. What does that mean to you?

Deidre: Butter has too many calories, and I'd feel too indulgent, and you're not supposed to eat butter on a diet. Lowering calories means I'll lose weight.

Me: I have the medical release form issued by your doctor, and there was nothing that indicated any nutritional restrictions. Did your doctor say anything to you that would cause you to feel medically concerned about eating it?

Deidre: No. Actually, my cholesterol level is in the normal range.

Me: Would you have assigned a different preference number if you added some butter?

Deidre: I'd love that. It's funny, but as soon as I thought about butter on my hot cereal, I began to crave it.

Me: Loving something to the point of craving it describes a "five" preference.

Deidre: With butter it would absolutely be a five preference.

Me: Just a suggestion, but I'm wondering how it would feel if you added a little butter? Maybe you'd lose weight a little more slowly, but it would have been "a five-preference" entry.

Deidre: This is the first time I'm being told to eat more, and it feels awesome. Absolutely!

Me: You might want to consider losing weight at a slower pace if it means giving yourself permission to eat "five-preference" foods. Choosing foods you love while losing or maintaining your weight means you can probably eat that way for the rest of your life.

HUNGER COLUMN

Me: I see you wrote down a "three" in the hunger column for this entry. How did you come up with this number?

Deidre: To be honest, I was very confused about this column. My stomach was rumbling, so I knew I needed to eat.

Me: When your stomach makes sounds, you interpret that as hunger?*

*There are many physical sensations people assume to be an indication of hunger, and stomach rumbling is one of them. Stomach rumblings are natural sounds associated with digestion and metabolism of food. Sensations around the stomach area have nothing whatsoever to do with hunger; but for now with regard to filling in the hunger column, do the best you can. A very specific exercise is included in Chapter 16 that will allow you to figure out what hunger actually is.

Deidre: Yes.

Me: I'm wondering, what would have happened if you had waited to eat?

Deidre: I couldn't wait any longer, since I had to get to work.

Me: What happens if you get too hungry?

Deidre: I get very nervous, headachy, and usually end up eating everything in sight. If I didn't eat then, I didn't know when I'd get a chance to eat again, and it might have been too late in the afternoon.

Me: I'm wondering if what you're calling a "three" hunger includes reactions in anticipation of the possibility of getting too hungry. Your mind is telling you, "I better eat something now." I'm also wondering whether this assessment of hunger may include some anxiety.

Deidre: I do get very nervous at the thought of where or when my next meal will be, and I think that this might have been the case.

Me: If you were a woman of leisure and had all the time in the world, and if with a snap of your fingers you would be brought food, could you have easily not eaten at that moment?

Deidre: Yes. On weekends I eat a lot later. If I didn't have to go to work this morning, I could have easily not eaten.

Me: I'm crossing out the "three" hunger.

Deidre: I really wrote down a "three" hunger?

Me: Yes, an indication that you needed to eat then and waiting any longer would mean you waited too long to eat.

Deidre: Well, I think I could have easily waited an hour or two, but the more I think about it, I was a *little* hungry.

Me: That's describes a "one" hunger perfectly, so I'll write that in your hunger column.

Deidre: So you're saying if I wasn't hungry, I shouldn't be eating?

Me: Not at all. All we're doing here is correcting your assessment of the different levels of hunger. We're going to be repeatedly revising information recorded in your ledger. The goal is learning how to accurately assess hunger versus appetite. When that distinction is made, you'll become more objective about your food choices. In the following months, you'll be researching "zero" hunger entries. It will become apparent that entries of "zero" hunger require different decision-making patterns, because eating whether hungry or not will never be a measurement of weight-loss success or failure.

Leaving no empty columns *before* eating is what will enable you to pay more accurate attention to physical sensations coming from your body. For the next several weeks, we're going to be changing most of your hunger numbers anyway, so for now, estimate what you think your hunger is, and write that number in the hunger column. Just do the best you can. Success at the end of the first month includes differentiating physical sensations that aren't hunger. It will take a while before you'll be able to figure out what hunger sensations actually are.

Deidre: Okay. There are a few diets that suggested writing down food intake, but this is different. I now sort of understand how you want me to use the ledger, and I love the whole experience. But this is the first time that I'm being told to write down data beforehand, and I really don't fully understand how it works.

Me: A lot of information has been gathered so far, and this one entry has told us a great deal about your current eating habits. Addressing one entry at a time is the most effective way to recall data and not feel overwhelmed. So in order to avoid feeling overwhelmed, this is as far as we'll go today. After Friday's appointment, you'll have a much better handle on how the ledger is used.

DISCUSSION

From a learning perspective, behavioral changes are effectuated by making the paired association between specific eating patterns and data derived from the scale. The ledger is what provides a simple and accurate data-gathering experience. Again, visible behaviors are controllable. A "pre-entering" system enables thinking about a behavior before actually exhibiting it. This will become the most effective way to shape new productive and goal-oriented behaviors. The act of entering data into the ledger comprises the cognitive/behavioral model that assumes people who learn to control their own behavior—more fundamentally, those learning to have confidence in the ability to control their own behavior—are much more likely to avoid an unrecoverable relapse.

CALORIES

Calories are also an easy way to quantify food-related data. In order to weigh less, you'll have to lower your caloric intake. Historically, dieters have used the scale and calories as the method for differentiating what they should and shouldn't consume. As advocated by Dr. Lulu Hunt Peters more than a century ago, the daily calorie ceiling people should target is approximately twelve hundred calories.

Like most, Deidre will be inclined to follow a target of twelve hundred calories per day. As previously indicated, while the ICP does have a caloric component to it, it is *not* a calorie-counting program in the traditional sense. Helping clients get away from imposing a fixed caloric ceiling has always included willpower. Getting away from daily caloric restrictions has proven to be the most demanding adjustment for veterans of other dieting regimes during the first few weeks of treatment in the ICP.

Assessing calories will become a component in the measurable data used to identify experiences that contribute to consistent and inconsistent goal-achievement thinking and acting. Calorie counting will slowly segue from a complex array of regimented eating behaviors associated with the external food rules of a diet into a more internalized guide for the voluntary monitoring of your eating choices and for determining whether or not your needs are being met. In the following chapter, we will learn how to fine-tune caloric manipulation. This is the only method for researching how to effectively use food to self-soothe while concurrently having a successful weight-loss experience.

HUNGER

There are neurons that send chemical signals throughout our body and bring information to the brain, causing other cells to take information away from the brain. All these cells communicate with each other via electrical fields. The biological need to eat (hunger) derives from glucose deficits and stimulates different degrees of physical reactions, causing generalized feelings of hunger from the lateral hypothalamus and generating sensations throughout the body.

What we experience as hunger are physical sensations emanating from signals in the cells of our body through what's called a synapse. Charles S. Sherrington coined this word in 1897. The word originates from the Greek words *synaptein* (to fasten together) and *haptien* (to fasten).

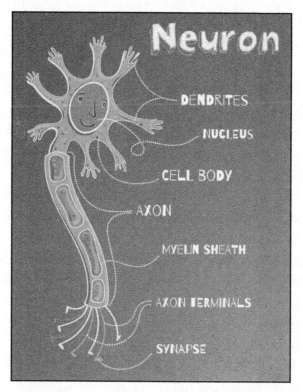

What hunger looks like on a cellular level in our body:

An electrical current travels from the dendrite down to the axon of one cell. Electrical information is conveyed to another cell close by. This is called an electrical synapse. Information to the hunger center of our brain is based on this electrical messaging system causing motivation that is experienced as an eagerness to eat. True hunger is the result of nutritional factors that consist mainly of blood glucose surging throughout our circulatory system. The hunger equation is: Nutritional deficits stimulate a need to eat. As we eat, blood glucose surges throughout our body. After about twenty to thirty minutes, our body regains specific blood-glucose levels that result in a state of homeostasis or normal equilibrium. Naturally thin people eat when hungry and stop when full.

Due to the fact that electrical synapses never shut down, we are continually being bombarded with physical sensations as a result of the constant firing of electrical charges throughout our body. Most physical sensations felt within our body—from salivation in our mouth to feelings above the pubic bone—have nothing whatsoever to do with hunger. In the majority of cases, our body is triggered to respond to environmental cues from whatever is going on around us.

Most often, obese people have learned early on that food produces a state of well-being, however illusory, and that failing to react to physical and environmental stimuli by not eating may lead to more negative feelings, such as anxiety and depression. They learn (in many cases as children) to use eating to bring about temporary positive feelings and to avoid experiencing emotional pain.

Motivation to resolve issues through eating, while short-lived, can alleviate tension and restore a seeming sense of emotional equilibrium. Overweight people are predisposed to deal with their feelings of shame by eating when they are not hungry. Scientific studies have proven that food in the mouth does produce anesthetic-type qualities of relief from stress, depression, and anxiety and that eating is effective when it comes to self-soothing.

The equation is quite simple: if you are hungry, eat; if you are not hungry, don't eat. If you're not hungry, it's also okay to eat. *The trick is to know the difference!* The ICP takes off where all diets leave you—it shows how to eat when you're not hungry and still lose or maintain your weight. Eating at a "zero" hunger level must be normalized. *Learning how to decipher different types of physical cues for what motivates eating behaviors is the key.* Making the distinction between needing to eat (hunger) versus wanting to eat (appetite) opens up research options as a way to reevaluate food choices and patterns.

I tell Deidre that by the third month she'll feel confident she's acquiring pragmatic skills for self-soothing with food while still working toward her weight-loss goal. Once understood, this information goes a long way toward helping one appreciate his or her learned eating patterns. Learned patterns result in habits. Habits may be defined as behaviors that, when frequently repeated, become automatic. (James 1899.) Through the application of both principles integral to the ICP (i.e., not eating the contract food and preconsumption ledger keeping), you'll begin to measure success by increasing the frequency of eating when hungry while decreasing the frequency of eating when not hungry. If you're not hungry but want to eat (for whatever reason), you'll know exactly how to do so, while still working toward attaining your goal.

Next I tell Deidre to accept the fact that, for now, she probably has no realistic idea of what hunger is but that by consistently using the hunger and preference columns in her ledger, she will eventually be guided toward learning how to assess physical sensations that indicate hunger. Assigning how much you like a food on a scale from one to five is the easiest way to distinguish between needing versus wanting to eat. Assigning different enjoyment qualities to each item means tackling a decision-making problem.

PREFERENCE

This is the most important column for the first week or two, since the number-one priority is not focusing on hunger but learning how to use your body as a barometer (the measurement of physical changes) and appropriately respond to external cues. Since it's effortless to pick out how much an orange or a baked potato is enjoyed compared with a radish or a beet, assigning an accurate likeability quotient will provide immediate feedback concerning what you're about to eat. A sense of confidence in this number interrupts feelings of shame that have always been associated with how enjoyable food is.

The most powerful way to benefit from the preference column is to insist that *once a preference number is assigned to any item, it becomes its permanent number*. While it may seem unimportant, the preference is categorized as an object constant. Anytime you attach an object constant to any behavior (especially those that are food related), you can rely on one specific measurement that becomes a personalized frame of reference for comparing how to make the distinction between the need versus the desire to eat.

Comparing different foods helps categorize and prioritize foods that might better meet weight-loss or maintenance goals. The ease of using this column provides an immediate sense of control regarding the choice of a food item. As trivial as it might seem, a constant preference number is the simplest and most effective means for counter-conditioning feelings of shame, confusion, and anxiety when it comes to every food choice. This provides the window for making transitions from external to internal cues.

Before ending our session, I pose a question to Deidre about her experience of our session.

> *Deidre*: I've kept food diaries before, but this one is different. I understand now how to do the ledger, and I love the whole ICP experience so far. This is the first time that I'm being told to eat more if I want to. Still, as I said before, I really don't fully understand how it works. But I imagine a fuller understanding will come in time.

> *Me*: It will. Every time you leave my office, you'll have more information than when you came in. I'm confident that after Friday's appointment, this method will seem a lot more manageable.

> *Deidre*: I can appreciate that after what I've learned during today's session.

> *Me*: This entry in the preference column addresses everything you need to know so you can proceed on course until Friday's session. There was a great deal of analysis about the information recorded in your ledger, and because I don't want you to feel overwhelmed, this is as far as we will go today. What's most important is that by the end of the first week, automatic hand-to-mouth eating will be gone.

REVIEWING OUR MEETING

Wednesday's appointment is considered a success if Deidre walks away with a sense that we're moving forward with a data-collection process we both agree on. What's most significant is that she did not eat her contract food and was 100 percent compliant about writing down her food before consumption. All that's needed at this point is to help her make the correlation that she's proven herself capable of carrying out a particular behavior or course of action. While reliance on the scale is and always will be needed as an accurate and objective measurement of body weight, systematic analysis of her ledger will be the most effective way to ultimately break the hold that the scale has on her.

It takes effort to lose weight. Developing the requisite skills to maintain the weight lost will also take a considerable expenditure of effort that, at times, may seem futile. Why? Because succumbing to a temptation is a setback from which you've probably historically never been able to fully recover. The next chapter continues the analysis of Deidre's ledger in subsequent sessions, with the objective of attaining the ultimate goal of the ICP: to never again have to rely on willpower to manage food temptations.

14

◆

THE THIRD SESSION—THE FIRST "UH-OH" MOMENT

Deidre's story shares a key common denominator with the stories of her dieting brethren: the phenomenon of the dreaded unrecoverable relapse. It's important to keep in mind there is a 100 percent probability that, during all weight-loss attempts, all dieters will be enticed to go off track from their designated food plan.

The first nonadherent act is different for everyone, but it is actually identical in that it's anxiety provoking and challenging to a person's commitment to his or her current weight-loss attempt. Deidre's "uh-oh" moment, the source of the inevitable demise of every previous diet she tried, had always been attributable to the infamous Pink Box.

CORRELATION DOES NOT IMPLY CAUSATION

The ICP methodology involves a systematic analysis of each and every behavior, which promotes the opportunity for self-reflection. This is the pivotal difference between the ICP and other weight-loss methods. The ability to make connections and access the underlying reasons for why we do what we do is important and often leads to assumptions regarding causal correlations. But just because we know why we are eating the way we eat doesn't necessarily mean that we will make any changes. A successful recovery from a regression requires something more than mere insight.

Any real or perceived "oops" or deviation away from your eating plans must be dealt with swiftly and effectively. The following entry opens the door for Deidre to research and acquire the skills that will enable her to do exactly what she needs to do for a successful recovery each time she feels that she's gone off track. The focus is on the role self-observation plays when the decision-making process is involved. Establishing a link with how Deidre perceives her eating patterns is a central element in the process, and this can be be made apparent by analyzing one entry in her ledger. This systematic examination will bring Deidre face-to-face with the true cause of all her past weight-loss failures.

This will be expeditiously accomplished because the ICP introduces a reinforcement or support schedule that is much more effective for lifelong weight management than dieting and more powerful than the immediate gratification of food. This is, in effect, the Holy Grail that the ICP provides—namely, the ongoing state of conscientiousness at the moment of consumption.

As has been repeatedly underscored, making food choices consistent with goal achievement is contingent on the transition from external to internal strategies. Based on attribution theory (ascribing causal factors), there's a natural inclination to overvalue personality-based explanations for behaviors (thoughts such as: "I'm weak, lazy, lack willpower, and lack self-control") while undervaluing situational explanations for why we make the kinds of decisions we do when it comes to food choices (such as: smelling bacon or fresh-baked cookies, realizing it's lunchtime, having to eat this meal Mom made or risk hurting her feelings, etc.).

If we rely on positive and goal-consistent, internally based factors, it's more likely we'll experience a successful outcome, whereas responding to external factors contributes to uncontrollable responses that predispose us for failure. Management of these often competing and confounding attributions will be accomplished through the analysis of the entries in Deidre's ledger.

END OF FIRST WEEK—THE THIRD SESSION

It's Deidre's third appointment and the second time we will be meticulously examining her ledger entries. Always keep in mind that losing weight during the first few weeks is the most substantive predictor of future success, and therefore the ICP has been deliberately designed to practically guarantee success from the start of the program. That said, ironically, the most successful candidates in this method initially resort to following the food rules that initially worked for them in the past. Based on her past dieting experiences, Deidre is confident she already knows exactly what's required for cutting back on food intake in order to lose weight.

At the beginning of the ICP, I make it a point to neither encourage nor discourage clients from resorting to whatever actions they deem necessary to shed pounds. As far as Deidre is concerned, she's primed to comply with dieting rules that have always initially worked for her in her past, convinced they'll surely be successful this time around. Of course, I realize that she's deluding herself and that these eating behaviors obviously have never worked over the long haul. The evidence of their failure is that she's sitting in my office and is incrementally being exposed to a new methodology for losing weight and managing weight loss. I refrain, however, from confronting her with this fact.

The next several sessions are intended to prepare her for the first time that the scale goes up, which will inevitably happen. This is the exact moment that historically indicated the beginning of the end for her previous dieting efforts and signaled a potential irreversible falling off the wagon phenomenon (i.e., an unrecoverable relapse). In comparison to her previous diets, however, this is the exact moment when the ICP shines through the gloom and doom. Adherence to both fundamental precepts of the ICP—not eating her contract item and completing her ledger before eating—are designed to enable Deidre to experience a sense of *behavioral integrity* about her food choices that will sustain her ongoing motivation and goal orientation despite any temporary setback the scale provides.

The following section addresses what Deidre experienced as an "oops" moment or, in the case of the ICP, a technical hiccup. The technical hiccup is the result of how she responded to the very first time she entered a piece of data in a column in her ledger that, in her mind, was wrong. In her previous weight-loss attempts, doing something perceived as wrong forced Deidre to return to a hypervigilant state when it came to adhering to food choices. Doing something wrong was anxiety provoking. Feelings of being back in control wouldn't be restored until she regained hypervigilance, which would provide her with confidence that she was back on track and following her prescribed food rules. Still, given her proclivity for hypervigilance, she would never feel complete confidence from that point forward. As a consequence of her misstep, her negative ruminations about making a mistake and the anticipation of future failures were constantly on her mind. Such thoughts functioned as a potential precipitating event that could lead to a permanent relapse and abandonment of the program.

Today's session brings to light what is going on in Deidre's mind about what constitutes a mistake. In contrast to every weight-loss attempt in her past, she will leave my office today with one key insight: while they are distractions to her sense of well-being, mistakes are simply data that must be investigated. The bad news is that as a consequence, Deidre's confidence is significantly, albeit temporarily, compromised.

The good news is that making her "oops" highly visible and helping her develop skills for handling it will establish the pattern for how she'll view the ledger from this point on. The methodical analysis of a behavior that caused her to feel bad and that would have previously signaled the beginning of the end of her efforts to lose weight will actually end up causing her confidence to skyrocket.

GOAL SEEKING SUSTAINS MOTIVATION

The ICP methodology of systematically recording and analyzing eating behaviors makes visible the information that enables you to learn from your experiences. Most importantly, it provides a means to help you make changes congruent with your weight-loss goal.

Deidre is already beginning to understand that she's the one responsible for all her food choices. Other than not eating her contract food, she's not being told what she should or shouldn't eat. She's not going hungry, so there's no need for her to exert willpower or self-control. And the scale is still going down. She mentions, "For the first time in my life, I'm not dieting to lose weight." Feelings of comfort surface almost immediately, and she declares: "The ICP is nothing like I've ever done."

For all these reasons, Deidre's desire to comply is getting stronger the more she sees herself benefitting from the program and the more she has personal involvement in producing the results she's looking for. Granted, it's virtually impossible not to engage old habits from the past, but that's becoming less problematic, because she's not being told what to eat. It only took one time going over the ledger for Deidre to be thrilled by the way personal information (her data) was made available and usable. She began to view her entries with a sense of originality, prompting her to be motivated to enlist a more "thinking for myself" mentality—the foundation for developing productive self-reflection strategies.

All this is in preparation for encouraging an honest and authentic internal dialogue that addresses her current eating patterns. The experience of adherence to both rules of the ICP is helping elicit a heightened *internal awareness* process concerning her food choices. Self-awareness promotes evaluating the decision-making required to make sure one's needs are being met and provides the foundation for feelings of self-control.

Seeing the tangible effects of her ledger is becoming an invaluable asset for Deidre. While her attachment to her ledger is growing, her performance anxiety is also increasing. The following interaction describes the pivotal moment when her anxiety surfaces due to an indicated noncompliant entry. It represents the first time Deidre feels she did something wrong.

The error is an example of a nonadherent-type entry. Many people would see this type of mistake as inconsequential and void of any need to react emotionally when the behavior was pointed out. The matter would be addressed briefly, and we'd proceed.

In Deidre's case, she had a profound adverse emotional reaction to being responsible for the nonadherent-type entry. Many of my clients often purposefully choose not to attend to these negative feelings at first, so they're kept safely under the radar. I realized, however, that given Deidre's reaction, had I allowed her journal entry to go unexamined, it would have jeopardized her future success in the ICP. The way in which the flawed entry was handled is described below.

FRIDAY'S SESSION

As we walk toward my office, Deidre confirms that she's been 100 percent faithful in completing her ledger. There are no empty columns, and she wrote everything down before eating. She gets on the scale. It shows she's down another one-and-a-half pounds, making a total of five pounds since Monday. Again, people who have had a significant weight gain before beginning the ICP most often show a dramatic weight loss in the first week or two. As previously pointed out, this is based on the fact that over 90 percent of foods are sodium bearing, so cutting back and changing some food choices even a little will release a lot of water at first.

At least 70 percent of weight reduction is water weight during the first several weeks. After that, people start to lose weight more slowly. There's a big difference between water loss and actual adipose (fat) loss, a key distinction not indicated by the scale.

After we sit down, I ask Deidre what it's been like not eating her contract food. She indicates that she's been fanatical about not wanting to come close to anything chocolate. She describes that when seeing a chocolate chip cookie commercial Monday night, she actually ran out of the room. By Wednesday, she remained in the room when this commercial was playing, but she closed her eyes and put her hands over her ears and started humming.

When asked if it took willpower or self-control to do so, she smiles and replies, "That's the weird part. It wasn't willpower at all but something else. I made a contract with you and we shook hands to solidify it. I really don't know what it was, but it was a lot easier than I thought it was going to be. It actually feels like an accomplishment not having eaten chocolate since Monday. Looking back now, it's funny when I remember how I jumped off the sofa and ran out of the room that first night."

The following entries in her ledger include the dinner entry from the night before. After her eleventh day, Deidre has followed the ICP 100 percent.

Time	Activity/Location	Food/Portion	Calories	Hunger*	Preference*
6:18	Rest. with friend	Salad	50	?*	5
		2 tbsp. dressing	160		5
		6 oz. salmon	300		5
		Iced tea w	0		5
		1 slice lemon	2		5

SEEKING TRUTH CAN BE A HEAVY BURDEN

The journey toward uncovering our true nature regarding food is challenging, especially when it entails helping people research behaviors they consider inconsistent with what they're trying to accomplish. Hence, it's important to make Deidre's ledger her friend and ally from the start. For this reason, the analysis starts by focusing on the most innocent-looking entry: the slice of lemon for two calories. Focusing attention on this entry first is certain to guarantee a sense of pride for Deidre. Indeed, she exudes satisfaction when describing how she came up with the calories and how meticulous her research was.

My acknowledgement of her obvious sense of integrity signifies my recognition of how aligned and compliant she is with the program. The precision of her lemon entry needs to be positively reinforced since, unbeknownst to her, we are about to explore an entry that is under her radar (but not mine).

Next, I ask Deidre about the question-mark entry. (From my clinical perspective, this represents the previously referred to nonadherent behavior.) She immediately goes into a defensive justification mode and exudes anxiety about her entry. Any paired association with her ledger and even the least amount of discomfort is indicative of a hiccup or a regression. She then describes how she didn't know her hunger level but didn't want to make a mistake by leaving an empty space.

As previously discussed, clients frequently come in with technical problems concerning the ledger during the first month of the program. A technical mishap is most often perceived as a minor irritant and doesn't usually trigger any feelings of discomfort. Clients come in for their appointments expressing a minimal amount of confusion and frequently want to discuss an entry or two. As far as they're concerned, their faith in the program or how they're doing hasn't been compromised.

This isn't the case with Deidre's question-mark entry. Specifically, the "I didn't want to make a mistake" comment was a red flag similar to what everyone experiences during the first month of treatment. Yet Deidre did not perceive it as a simple technical mistake; rather, it was quite anxiety producing for her.

Deidre's need to justify this entry was all the proof I needed for correlating and attuning a more apt emotional response to her technical deviation. By putting down my pen and notepad, I communicated to her that this entry was a cause for pause.

Something happens to everyone at some point during the first few weeks of any weight-loss program that brings up feelings of not meeting an expectation. When we are on a diet, what the scale indicates has always been the measurement of success or failure. The scale not budging or heaven forbid, going up, has classically been the first anxiety-provoking, irrefutable proof that we have made "bad" food choices.

In Deidre's case, her question mark had nothing to do with what food choice she had made or even with the scale. Rather, it was indicative in her mind of her consistent self-defeating actions that signified feelings of low self-esteem and inadequacy. Instead of making a bad food choice, writing down a question mark was Deidre's way of indicating confusion about how to accurately assess her hunger at that time. Her experience of technical inaccuracy with the ledger caused stress and feelings of emotional chaos.

At this moment, it's impossible for Deidre to appreciate the profound insight she's about to acquire by exposure to a recovery process that focuses on using her seemingly innocuous question-mark entry as a springboard. Nitpicking her question mark is what will lead her on the path to appreciating the importance of technical accuracy when it comes to ledger keeping.

Deidre is about to identify the root cause for every one of her past weight-loss failures: missed expectations. The motivation to meet expectations and the fear of ultimately (and inevitably) missing them forced her to enlist coping strategies as a way to manage the ensuing feelings of discomfort. Ideally, she'll begin to apply this eye-opening insight to every other decision-making area in her life.

The theme for most people becomes not meeting expectations regarding food choices. Many decisions about eating behaviors are the result of not wanting to disappoint others. Over time, it becomes a well-ingrained habit.

Today, I come right out and ask: "How did you learn how to meet others' expectations?"

Tears begin to well up in Deidre's eyes.

Deidre: My dad's from France. His culture and upbringing taught him that being thin is an indication of self-control and self-respect. When he met my mom, she was just finishing up a medical fasting program and was very thin. Soon after marriage, she got pregnant with me and gained a lot of weight that she never lost. Dad had obvious disdain for my mom's weight, but I knew his love for me. He often reminded me that I also had his genes, so it was possible for me to lose weight. I just now realized that every time I dieted, it was really for my dad. It was important to meet his expectations, and obviously I always failed. Failing on all my diets meant I failed him.

Me: I'm curious; what was it like for you at the moment you wrote down the question mark?

Deidre: I wanted to please you and not leave any empty space, but honestly, it didn't feel good. Deep down I knew it was wrong.

Me: Did you believe that not writing down a number in the hunger column might influence your future success?

Deidre: Absolutely.

Me: What happened just prior to writing down the question mark?

Deidre: I just remembered something. I knew the waiter was busy, but wanting to make sure about my entry, I asked him how many calories were in the salmon I ordered. He was obviously bothered. He looked straight at me, rolled his eyes, and said he'd have to check. It made me feel terrible.

Me: What did his eye-rolling signify about you personally?

Deidre: He saw how fat I was, and I felt embarrassed and ashamed.

Me: If you had to put a feeling on a bumper sticker, what's the one feeling you're having right now in this room?

Deidre: Pissed.

Me: Writing in a question mark was anxiety provoking. Even in this short amount of time, you're obviously benefitting from doing the ledger. It took an act of significant aggression to give yourself permission to deviate from the protocol and do what you felt was wrong. I'm wondering: pre-ledger days, what would this have meant?

Deidre: To be completely honest, the way I felt, there was no way I could ever face you again, and that would have been the end of my diet.

Me: Have you thought about possibly not coming in?

Deidre: No—not for one moment.

Me: Remember, all we're doing is collecting incoming data, information about your entries and outgoing data, understanding from the information supplied. Whether perceived or actual, mistakes made during the first month are what we're investigating. For everyone, the hunger column is the most demanding and confusing component during the first several weeks. There are so many things that contribute to eating that have nothing to do with hunger. It's really hard not to learn from this program. As long as you follow the protocol, you'll be confident that every entry leads toward becoming a skilled researcher.

Something happens around the third-month mark that leads to correcting your assessment of all the different elements that previously meant hunger. For now, all you can do is begin researching what hunger is *not!* For the next week, you should use the following behavior just before writing down your hunger number: point to where you feel hunger.

Deidre: Here (pointing right below her belly button).

Me: That's where most people point.

During thirty years of working with clients, whenever I've asked where people felt hunger, I've gotten one of three answers:

1. They point to the area directly beneath the collarbone.

2. They point to the upper chest.

3. They point to the abdominal area right above the pubic bone.

Me: Deidre, as an exercise, next week before you enter numbers in your hunger column, gently rest your hand where you feel hunger and say: "This is where I feel hunger, but it's not accurate." That's all. Then just write down the number that you think is correct. After the next few weeks, you'll begin to compare one hunger entry with another. It's different for everyone, but it will take anywhere between three to perhaps six months or even a year before you'll have confidence in your assessment of what hunger actually is. For now, guess and do the best you can.

DISCUSSION

When it comes to following rules on a food plan, even the mere thought of possibly not meeting expectations is typically traumatic for dieters. All food decisions are scrutinized as a way to meet the expectations of the particular methodology being followed. In Deidre's case, the rules also had to be followed to prevent being criticized by the specter of her now-deceased dad.

Deidre's fierce loyalty and allegiance to her dad's expectations set her up to fail as soon as she deviated from what she knew must be done if she wanted to lose weight. It was critically important to help her make this connection. Writing down a question mark in her ledger had reduced her anxiety for a moment, since, as far as she was concerned, the column wasn't empty. She was trying to be a good and obedient girl.

Deidre began to appreciate that purposely choosing not to make an educated guess only magnified the fact she wasn't showing the level of technical integrity her ledger deserved. Helping put that behavior into perspective was important in that it showed her:

- How current ideas are learned and supported by previous experiences.

- That personal opinions come from fixed patterns secured in our memory banks.

- That existing attitudes persist in a very selective way and support an already intact belief system.

Deidre and other dieters have been programmed to believe that if they dare to deviate from their food plan, then they fail. At times, they might be forced to rely on their ability to invoke willpower and/or self-control to forestall potential problems. This strategy might prove successful at the onset of most weight-loss attempts. An unplanned eating event, however, usually makes the weight-loss goals unachievable.

Chapters 15 and 16 will continue to show how feelings coming from the salivary glands (on top of the jawbone) all the way down to the lower abdominal region have nothing to do with the biological state of hunger.

THE UH-OH MOMENT

The uh-oh moment in the world of dieting has always been managed based on a relapse-prevention model—an intervention model accepted in the medical community for all substance-use disorders. Under this model, relapse-prevention strategies are used to treat the addictive-type withdrawal and craving responses to highly preferable foods. For a dieter, any relapse-type behavior is the result of noncompliance with food rules, hence overeating occurs as a result of deviating from the diet's restrictions. People following any current weight-loss method will invariably break a rule, causing the "oops" feeling to surface. The relapse-prevention model views anyone who exhibits a food-related relapse (i.e., any deviation from the diet's food rules) as having reverted back to an earlier diseased state. If this occurs, the prognosis for recovery is poor. Thus, after any period of abstinence that is predicated on exerting unflagging willpower, a relapse must be prevented at all costs.

A key differentiating factor of the ICP is that it removes abstinence and self-imposed restraints when making food choices. Breaking the second ICP rule regarding ledger keeping means you didn't write down all the research characteristics of your eating behavior beforehand. The first rule is to not eat the contract food item. Neither rule requires you to resist the temptations of a wide variety of highly valued and pleasurable foods.

In contrast to a relapse-prevention model, any "oops" in the ICP will be dealt with based on what I've termed "recovery from a regression model." Instead of assigning an illness diagnosis to an overeating event, a regression is considered a trend or shift away from a goal. Eating patterns are seen as learned habits, whereby the ledger is a *pattern-recognition* tool that makes these behaviors highly visible. The process of making current patterns visible enables you to make changes consistent with your goal.

The recovery from a regression model will become a natural way of taking into account all food-related events that come into question. Applying this term (i.e., "recovery from a regression"), Deidre is about to incorporate what makes the ICP unique, and whenever an "oops" occurs, she'll have the requisite skills to make a full recovery by utilizing the ledger. Rather than producing shame, guilt, or anxiety, deviations become an opportunity for making better decisions about current food choices and open up options for making changes.

It's worth repeating: the extraordinary efficacy of the ICP that sets it apart from other programs is its capacity to decrease the frequency of regressions. Having a regression, paying attention to it, and getting back on track are considered predictable phenomena that can be strategically handled. This differentiates the ICP from any diet ever offered to the public. What's most noteworthy is that Deidre's lack of technical integrity was an internal process that had nothing to do with the scale, which is an external measurement of success or failure.

This model of recovering from a regression is one of the key focuses of the ICP. Categorizing an "oops"-type event as a regression enables you to successfully recover from these hiccups that will surely happen in the future.

15

◆

THE FOURTH WEEK—RECOVERY FROM REGRESSIONS AND THE MANAGEMENT OF CRAVINGS

MONDAY'S APPOINTMENT

This is the fourth week of the ICP for Deidre and her eighth appointment. As expected, she shows up on time. Her work schedule Monday through Friday is structured, making it much easier for her to control food choices on those days. Her weekends often involve less structure and more socializing, which can contribute to more unplanned eating events. For this reason, the appointment after the first weekend of using the ledger is especially significant.

Deidre has been inundated with loads of information that comprise the nuts and bolts of the "how-to-lose-weight" stage, and she has been performing admirably and doing exactly what she's been told to do. The principles of the ICP are sinking in. Since she's been making more thoughtful and productive food choices, she's more confident about how to go forward with the program.

As we walk toward my office, I ask how the program is going. Deidre confirms that she's been 100 percent on task when recording in her ledger, leaving no empty columns and writing down everything before consumption. We continue our small-talk ritual, and Deidre states how terrific she's been feeling. When she gets on the scale, she's down another three-quarters of a pound, making a total of four pounds since starting her program with me, and, of course, she's ecstatic.

Smiling, she quickly adds: "Yes, Deena, I'm getting enough food." She sits down and says, "I must tell you, the silliest thing happened this morning."

Deidre is about to tell me a story and disclose something that happened earlier that day. Any story about how the ICP has been applied suggests it's becoming an integrated personal experience. Deidre's role as a student dutifully following her teacher's guidelines is beginning to change, as it must so that she will become less dependent on me and more confident about the skills she's acquiring.

DEIDRE'S STORY—THE RAISIN

Deidre begins to describe how she felt like indulging in a little treat last night. Wanting to make her dinner a bit more special, she considered adding some raisins to her salad but hesitated because she felt a little uncomfortable. A nutritionist once told her to never mix fruit with vegetables, as it was shown that eating them together has a deleterious effect on how food is metabolized and could prevent weight loss.

> *Deidre*: From that point on, if I ever combined fruits with vegetables, I'd feel terrible. I felt that it was a sin to mix certain foods. But, nevertheless, I did something out of character last night. I began talking to myself, saying: "I'm not on a diet. Raisins aren't my contract food, and all I need to do is write them down in the ledger beforehand." I turned to the calorie app on my phone and saw small raisins are four calories each, and larger ones are five. Counting out fifteen raisins, I wrote down seventy-five calories in the calorie column and ate my salad. What felt especially good was that the raisins were obviously small, but I decided to account for them as being larger.

Everything was accurately accounted for before eating. It was the best salad I've ever eaten, and I still had a weight-loss day. But here's the silly part. On the way to work this morning, I noticed a single raisin on the kitchen counter that must have escaped my attention. I picked it up, walked over to the sink, and threw it down the garbage disposal.

Me: In pre-ledger days, what would you have done?

Deidre: Pop that sucker in my mouth without thinking twice.

Me: You didn't give up raisins, so what stopped you? Was it will-power?

Deidre: No, something else. Nobody was telling me *not* to eat it, so the decision was mine. The raisin was actually accounted for in my ledger last night. Still, I felt it would have to be accounted for this morning since the date, time, and hunger were different. All I needed to do was write it down. The ledger was in my purse. It didn't seem worth it to get my ledger out to write down one raisin.

Me: Hmm! It sounds as if writing in your ledger was more important than actually eating the raisin.

Deidre: I didn't think about that, but yeah, that's exactly right. I've never done anything like that before. In the past, there was always this sense of entitlement. If the raisin were on my food plan, I would still visit my inner brat who was always close by, egging me on. I would've seen that raisin as mine, and I would've deserved it. But I didn't have any of those feelings.

Me: Bottom line, what was that experience like for you?

Deidre: This is different than anything I've ever done. You weren't there last night telling me what I should or shouldn't eat. Whether I'm hungry or not, all I need to do is write in my ledger so that I'm on safe footing and never feel deprived. It's ironic, but I'm actually really enjoying food for the first time in my life. The question-mark entry I made three weeks ago didn't feel good, and I just don't want to play all the games I've played in the past. Something's changing.

I feel more grown up. It feels as if my "adult" has shown up and it's all up to me to keep her around. Throwing out that silly raisin proved I can do that.

Me: Throwing the raisin down the disposal couldn't serve as a better example of responsible behavior. Also, this kind of attention to eating behaviors most often results in losing weight. It appears as if you're beginning to cross over from goal achievement-type actions based on the scale toward actions based on consideration of what you need to do to achieve your weight-loss goal and stay there. The motivation to throw out the raisin was in no way correlated with the scale; it was something else. That something else is moving past losing weight as your only goal and is proof that you're starting to successfully research what's required to lose weight and sustain your weight loss. You deserve a legitimate attagirl: good job!

Deidre views integrity as her greatest asset. As previously discussed, her question-mark entry felt uncomfortable to her. In her mind, omitting the hunger number was unacceptable, since it represented a missed expectation concerning technical integrity. Therefore, the possibility of breaking the "leave no empty column" rule was resolved by writing down a question mark. Deidre's raisin story was an example of her integrity: she did not eat the raisin, because it wasn't written down in her ledger. Relating the story provided an opportunity for positive reinforcement of her greatest asset—integrity—and I seized upon it.

LEARNING OCCURS THROUGH PAIRED ASSOCIATIONS

There is a dynamic interplay between pleasurable foods and craving responses. An *association* between a food (stimulus) and eating (response) is contingent upon the food's *enjoyment quotient*. Highly enjoyable foods contribute to the development of personal eating patterns. This associative learning regarding food preferences is categorized as a *classically conditioned response*.

It's a simple formula. Any food we like, we'll want again. It's a scientifically proven fact that it only takes one paired association for a craving response to occur. For most, just thinking about a highly enjoyable food will trigger the desire for it. Triggered desires evoke automatic and reflexive-type responses. As long as a paired association exists, these kinds of responses can't be controlled. From the viewpoint of the medical model, if overeating episodes are not within our control, it's obvious why obesity has been categorized as incurable!

Just imagine the amount of incoming data we're continuously receiving. It's really quite a simple equation that determines whether an experience is retained in our memory or not. We break down information into small units so we can organize it better. That way, each experience can attach and integrate itself in a manner that's most effective for retrieval at a later time. But each and every event has the potential to be stored in our memory for long-term use or to be discarded; it all depends upon how our brain organizes the particular event.

A part of the brain called the *hippocampus* analyzes new input data and determines what's going to be done with it. The brain will strengthen, weaken, or destroy a thought, feeling, or behavior based on its worthiness for retention. Favorable reactions are reinforced; those deemed unfavorable are weakened. This is the basis for how all learning occurs.

RECOVERING FROM FEELINGS OF HOPELESSNESS

The first treatment principle of the ICP is *operant conditioning,* and it is learned, accessed, implemented, and practiced during the first month of treatment. "Operant" addresses the ways we *operate* in our environment. Writing down the food selected to be consumed beforehand is followed by the consequence, namely, the self-authorization to eat it. This consequence is a reaction to a sequential behavior that has a positive reinforcing effect. The act of writing in the ledger makes eating behaviors highly visible, and the high visibility of any behavior makes it more likely to be controllable and, hence, less automatic.

At the end of the first month's data gathering research experiment, a detailed map of current eating behaviors will evolve and become evident. Only then will it be possible to assure your success in making certain that food-related behaviors can be properly viewed and assessed objectively.

Implementing operant-conditioning methods for behavioral change will guarantee that you're able to benefit from the one core concept central to this book, namely, learning how to view eating behaviors objectively. It is imperative that you exhibit 100 percent compliance during the first month of this program. At the onset of any learning curve, compliant behaviors must be repeated over and over and over again. Only then will your newly found eating behaviors become a habit. The very structure of your conduct is the composite of the habits you form.

Habits formed from implementing the ICP are the result of researching solutions to determine what's best for you and how to implement the changes necessary to get your needs met. A willingness to accept frustrations as a normal part of your learning curve is imperative. There is a highly effective principle in psychology that will help you recover from any feelings of discomfort. It's called the "stop it" method. If you've done something that you consider counterproductive, all you need to say is, "Stop it" to yourself (out loud is best). This translates, for example, into taking a deep breath and picking up and weighing that banana you're about to eat. (By the way: Peeled bananas are thirty calories an ounce!) To illustrate this point, I want to share a personal experience.

One Tuesday eighteen years ago, at around 5:00 a.m., I was getting ready to drive the love of my life (my cowboy hubby, Paul…yes, I know this Brooklyn girl is attracted to cowboys) to the hospital for his long-overdue hip surgery. The day when he couldn't make it one block to our neighborhood store for a gallon of milk, he looked at me and said, "It's time."

I acquired my skills as a blood-gas technician when I worked part-time at UCLA while completing my dissertation in psychology. During surgery, when the measurement of blood-gas levels was required, it was a "stat" or emergency situation. The machines patients were hooked up to indicated when it was imperative to determine the oxygen level in their blood. These experiences prepared me to realize that potentially anything could go wrong while a patient was under anesthesia. The thought of possibly losing my husband evoked a terror that I'd never experienced.

Before I left for the hospital that morning, I remember going into the kitchen, peeling a banana, and putting it on the scale. It was 4.7 ounces. My terror was still with me, but the moment I wrote in my ledger (and before I ate the 141-calorie banana) I felt 100 percent in control.

Did my banana-eating behavior allay the thoughts of my husband dying on the operating table? No. While powerful, the ICP obviously can't miraculously stop all negative cognitions and emotions. But weighing my peeled banana and writing it down in my ledger before eating it afforded me a momentary sense of control. Albeit short-lived, that sense of control greatly subdued feelings of chaos.

In my pre-ledger days, at 220 pounds, I would have stopped on the way to the hospital to get a few breakfast sandwiches, an extra-large coffee with three-quarters cup of half-and-half and four packets of sugar, and a fried potato patty thrown in for good measure. Oh, I almost forgot the several packets of ketchup. During his surgery, I would have otherwise been wolfing down food—the one and only way I had learned to soothe my terror!

Having followed the ICP for over a decade at the time Paul had his surgery, it was possible for me to be 100 percent available for him when I was most needed. Rather than succumbing to shame and self-loathing, I was there for him before and afterward. That surgery gave me back my ski buddy! As I write this, we actually just returned from a ski trip to Mammoth Mountain. I call Paul my bionic skier on his titanium hip as we swoosh down the slopes together.

Ledger keeping makes positive and negative reinforcements observable. Positive reinforcements provide good feelings by encouraging certain behaviors. Negative reinforcements result in bad feelings. Behaviors that are positively reinforced get repeated until they become learned behaviors (i.e., habits).

Again, the ledger-keeping component of the ICP has been customized to make unthinking eating patterns highly visible. Successful compliance with the ICP protocol rests on learning how to go from unthinking consumption to conscientious eating. The only effective way to assure adherence at the onset is to provide a means to easily assess food-related thoughts and behaviors. Keep in mind that, although the ICP may appear to focus on the content of what's in the ledger, the real focus is on the process of how the information in the ledger is being used.

It is worth repeating that writing down what you intend to eat before-hand eliminates *automatic hand-to-mouth eating*. The ledger provides an ultimate sense of control by inhibiting the dynamic, spontaneous, and impulsive interplay between seeing food and eating it. By the end of the first month, Deidre is learning how to benefit from the data her ledger is providing. The more information acquired, the greater the confidence that there is a solution to the problem of being overweight. It's up to each individual to determine what solution works best.

The more confidence Deidre has in the program, the more likely her role in the current student-teacher relationship will begin to diminish. The painstaking analysis of the ledger will gradually make this increasingly independent state of mind a reality. During the first month, adherence to both rules of the ICP virtually guarantees successful weight loss. Ledger keeping becomes the way to initiate a new weight-loss mind-set.

The first month's focus is in preparation for that inevitable moment when it feels as if you've gone off track. While the question-mark entry caused Deidre to doubt her integrity, the raisin incident subsequently reaffirmed that integrity—and then some. When Deidre was following a traditional dieting program, the leading cause of an unrecoverable regression was the first time the scale went up. But with the ICP, everything about the first month has been to gear Deidre toward breaking the association between the scale, performance anxiety, and missed expectations.

The treatment phase for the first month continues to help Deidre make self-observations a positive experience. This will help extinguish resistance to the ICP protocol while enhancing compliance. The shift to acquiring self-monitoring skills will become the focus of attention as the most effective way to de-emotionalize past dieting experiences and to move Deidre away from dependence on the scale as the only measurement of success. The question is: what happens after the first month and every month afterward?

There's a downside to relying solely on ledger keeping for permanent habit formations: every ounce of control derived from recording data in a ledger has no effect on abating the craving response. Ledger keeping is based on operant conditioning. Current preferences based on eating habits are so ingrained and automatic that cravings can prevail over any habits learned during the first month of ledger keeping. Although recording in your ledger does magnify a sense of control, unfortunately, operant conditioning has minimal capacity to maintain feelings of control when it involves succumbing to a temptation (i.e., a craving response). And succumbing to a temptation is a hurdle that you've never been able to recover from in the past. Most regressions are the result of a spontaneous and unplanned eating event—an event that will undoubtedly occur in the future and result in feelings of anxiety.

It's time to state the second and last hypothesis of your experiment: *Adherence to both rules of the ICP—giving up one food item and ledger keeping—accomplishes not only weight loss but will also contribute to the development of strategies for weight-loss sustainability.*

The next chapter expands upon the discussion of the first scientific principle used in the ICP–*classical conditioning.* This principal propels the ICP beyond every other weight-loss program you've ever attempted. Specifically, the next chapter helps you to develop self-directedness by fostering positive behavioral outcomes based on the ongoing management and extinction of the craving response.

16

♦

SELF-DIRECTION

Self-knowledge is the key to self-modification. Your actions—behaviors, thoughts, and feelings—are embedded in situations, and each of these elements must be carefully observed. Self-observation is the first step on the road to self-directed behavior—and it is the step most often omitted in our daily lives. Most of us assume that we understand ourselves, and we rarely feel that we need to employ any systematic, self-observation techniques. But real surprises may be in store for the person who begins careful self-observation. Genuine discoveries are made.
—*Self-Directed Behavior*, Watson, David L., 1934

Since the turn of the last century, emotional and physical health has improved with the help of experimental psychologists. The main focus of attention is how to help people enlist self-directed behaviors as a way to improve their quality of life. Laboratory and field research have made tremendous headway within the healthcare fields. As an example, patients' adherence to self-care protocols leads to decreased doctor visits and shortened time spent in hospitals. But there's one population that seems to be benefitting the least from all the self-directed behavioral research: those with weight-related issues.

Problems arise not because dieters aren't able to enlist self-directed strategies, but because traditional dieting regimes force dieters to abide by this rule: when hungry, eat; when sated, stop. Eating for any other reason than being hungry is considered taboo, an offense that must be avoided at all costs. For this reason, dieters are coerced into eating only when hungry and coerced to enlist a "firmness of mind" attitude to manage and control non-hunger-eating episodes. This imposed mind-set is best described as exerting willpower, which includes:

1. Self-discipline.

2. Self-control.

3. Determination.

WILLPOWER

There will be some point when dieters will be forced to rely on willpower as a way to put off or delay unwanted eating events.

In the weight-loss field, the so-called experts who specialize in self-management skills view willpower as muscle building—the more it's used, the stronger it gets. Willpower aficionados believe that the use of willpower will help activate impulse-control strategies that can be employed whenever needed.

Granted, in the early stage of losing weight, it's somewhat effortless to eat only when hungry; but, eventually, the infamous nonhunger eating episodes begin to occur. Yet all the willpower we're able to muster isn't strong enough to overcome a craving response. When a craving does happen, the experts believe motivation to lose weight compels the dieter into relying on willpower as the ultimate way to adhere to the rules.

It turns out that relying on willpower as a way to avoid dieting failures is merely a temporary fix. Depending on it as a fix for the long haul will be fruitless. It's clear that a long-term substitute for willpower is vital if weight loss is to be sustained and craving impulses are to be managed.

THE BEHAVIORAL LANGUAGE OF INTROSPECTION

Taking the first step toward self-directed eating behavior requires the ability to feel that it's normal to eat for reasons besides hunger. The opportunity for implementing self-directed actions begins by assuming a noncritical attitude and normalizing nonhunger-eating events. As previously indicated, the ICP is based on operant and classical conditioning principles that provide the opportunity for self-directed behavioral skills without ever having to rely on willpower.

Operant techniques are based on the idea that if a behavior is rewarded with a perceived pleasant consequence, the behavior is more likely to be repeated and become constant. A consequence is a reaction to a behavior that serves as a reinforcement. The consequence of self-recording data—feelings, associated cognitions, and behaviors surrounding eating patterns—makes behaviors observable. Visibility provides impetus for self-understanding and a greater feeling of being in control, leading to self-management-type actions.

Discernible behaviors promote objective and logical decision-making. Logical thinking diminishes feelings of anxiety. Less anxiety makes one more emotionally and physically resistant to the knee-jerk of environmental cues, such as TV ads featuring chocolate chip cookies or candy. But it's still not possible or realistic to stop turning to food as a way to self-soothe. If nonhunger eating can never be eliminated, how can one ever lose and keep weight off permanently? The answer is: a successful weight-loss program requires decreasing the frequency and caloric magnitude when these episodes inevitably occur.

The next and last chapter describes the only way this can be accomplished. You already have a working knowledge of the second principle of the ICP, the operant approach by employing ledger keeping. The following discussion focuses on the first principle—classical conditioning. Compliance with both principles makes it possible to verify the final hypothesis of your research: *Adherence to the ICP protocol accomplishes not only weight loss but will also contribute to the development of strategies for weight-loss sustainability.* Working side by side, these two scientific principles will enable you to manage all the nonhunger eating events that will surely occur in your future.

Classical conditioning is best described by considering circumstances where highly preferred foods elicit a craving response. Food cravings evoke powerful emotional and physical reactions that, heretofore, have been considered uncontrollable. Relying on Pavlov's salivary extinction model, any food item given up will cause a reduction and, eventually, an extinction of the bodily and emotional desire (i.e., craving response) for that food. Note that an added benefit during the period of a fading craving response is that bodily sensations and emotional states will become more discernible.

The ICP uses a classical conditioning approach by giving up one out-of-control food item, the contract food. Once a powerful eating cue, our contract food becomes something we are less and less interested in. Decon-ditioning the desire for one food item creates powerful effects on a person's patterns of thinking and feeling. The "lessening of the desire" phase supports a meaningful and structural insight into the workings of the inner self.

For Deidre, this became more and more noticeable when we observed that most of her food-related anxieties were being replaced with a profound sense of accomplishment. She'd go to bed each night assured by one irrefut-able fact: "I haven't eaten my contract food." Introspection and choice, rather than willpower, became the foundation for changing her eating patterns.

LOSING WEIGHT WREAKS HAVOC ON THE BODY

The more one loses weight, the greater one's feelings of vulnerability. This is the point when people begin to complain about having butterflies in their stomach, shaking all over, and feeling a sense of breathlessness. Some start to have aches, pains, and nausea. During this weight-loss phase, high stress exaggerates one's mental and bodily reactions to it. These heightened reac-tions happen at some point for virtually everyone.

For Deidre, her heightened reactions begin about three months into the program. Not having to invoke willpower to avoid self-soothing with food magnifies her emotional and physical reactions. She begins to pay more attention to her physical sensations. On one occasion, she describes watching TV at night when all of a sudden she notices her heart beating during an especially exciting moment, and she finds it hard to breathe. Like many of those who preceded her in the ICP, Deidre begins to claim during this time period that, in some ways, she feels worse now than she had before starting the program. Then it happened.

THE THIRD MONTH

Around her three-month mark, Deidre shows up for a scheduled Monday appointment. She tells me that something happened the previous Friday that she needs to talk about. Her boss, normally a mild-mannered person, is under a lot of stress. Deidre recounts, "It was an innocent oversight on my part, but still he yelled at me in front of my colleagues. Feeling terribly embarrassed, I made a decision right then and there to have a special treat for lunch. My thought was: 'I'm feeling bad, and I want to feel better; I want a burger.' I'd been thinking about it for a while, but still, it was unplanned. In the old days, eating at the burger joint while trying to lose weight would be unheard of. It meant my diet was over."

> *Deidre continues*: You told me specifically not to change anything I'd do normally. I decided to go to my favorite burger joint for my favorite meal—burger, fries, and a shake. While at my desk at work, I opened up my ledger and looked up everything on the calorie app on my phone. Here's what I wrote down:

Time	Activity/Location	Food/Portion	Calories	Hunger*	Preference*
1:18	Mel's Burgers	4 oz. meat	320	3	5
		Bun	220		
		Small fries	230		5
		8 packs ketchup	120		
		Small vanilla shake	400		5

Previously, I'd go hog wild by ordering a double burger with double cheese and extra special sauce, jumbo fries with lots of ketchup (maybe fifteen or twenty packets), and an extra-large chocolate shake. This time, eating at the burger joint was different. That's not to say there wasn't anxiety about what I was about to eat, but writing everything down beforehand helped manage many of those feelings. Stepping up to the counter, I ordered exactly what was written in my ledger. I got my order, sat down, and ate my lunch.

The food was delicious, and the fact is that while eating it I did feel better. I didn't stop feeling bad about the way my boss treated me, but it was the first time I wasn't feeling bad about my food. For the first time in my life, I didn't feel guilty afterward.

Pre-ledger days, a burger, fries, and a shake would have put me into binge mode. Instead, when I got home from work, I still felt stuffed. I ended up not eating any more that day—but not because of feeling bad and guilty about having gone off a diet. I chose not to eat any more because I was still stuffed. For the first time in my life, I had a taste of what it felt like to eat like a normal person, getting my needs met on all levels. I turned to some of my favorite foods as a way to feel better. Eating calmed me down, I didn't feel guilty, and I ended up still feeling on track toward my goals. I want more of that.

Lying in bed that night, it came to me: I listened to my body. Rather than feeling anxious and out of control, I relished the thought that the shake wasn't chocolate!

Me: I'm wondering, was it willpower or some other reason for not eating chocolate?

Deidre: Hmm! I just realized at this moment that willpower had absolutely nothing to do with it; actually, it was just the opposite. When ordering a vanilla shake, I smiled and felt terrific because I hadn't broken any rules. I really was looking forward to that shake. Having it actually helped me feel better about the rest of my lunch.

Until this incident, Deidre still had doubts that she'd be able to surpass the three-month mark. This was the point when she'd begin to experience her feelings more acutely. With every other weight-loss method, she felt nervous most of the time and felt vulnerable about the possibility of failing. The necessity to avoid the diet's taboo foods forced her to resort to will-power. Because it was impossible to contain intense emotional and physical states as they escalated during the weight-loss phase, she turned to one food in particular as a way to feel better: anything chocolate. Yet eating this food made her vulnerable to experiencing feelings of self-loathing.

With the ICP, not having her contract food and writing in her ledger activated a confidence Deidre had never experienced. Not eating chocolate was proof she had taken control of the one thing that had always meant a downfall leading to an unrecoverable relapse. She now realized that the experience of not eating chocolate provided the opportunity to investigate comparisons of her old eating patterns with her current and future food choices. Not eating chocolate had become the impetus for transforming an external reward (chocolate) into an internal reinforcement schedule (self-control).

Not consuming her contract food and using the ledger opened up the opportunity for Deidre to experience integrity about her choice for lunch. Positive feelings about the vanilla shake replaced feelings of guilt, precipitating something more powerful than the immediate gratification of chocolate—the power of a positive inner reinforcement schedule gained from *not* eating it. She began to get excited about the prospect of researching new ways to modify all her food-related decisions from that point onward.

Not eating your contract food supports the emotional and mental attitudes that help you stay on track despite stressful events. Together with ledger-keeping, salivary extinction of one food item will provide vital self-management skills during the weight-loss stage.

UNDERSTANDING SELF-PERCEPTION BASED ON ATTRIBUTION THEORY

A discussion about one's disposition includes frequently experienced moods inclining us to act in a particular way. These learned habits or tendencies can be measured with behavioral profiles taken from early childhood. Moods most often come about based on how people assign meaning for why things happen the way they do, which is a concept described as *attribution theory*. This theory addresses how people attribute causes for what happens in their lives. How one deals with the external world becomes correlated with self-perception.

An attribution for the cause of an event is comprised of three major elements:

1. Locus is the perceived location of the cause.

2. Stability describes whether the cause is perceived as static or dynamic over time.

3. Controllability describes whether a person feels actively in control of the cause.

All three elements play a role in how we perceive ourselves when it comes to meeting or not meeting expectations.

People with self-esteem issues are inclined toward making correlations that a job well done means they are a good person. They're also inclined to over-exaggerate mistakes and under-exaggerate accomplishments. When people attribute failures to stable factors (i.e., issues that are likely to recur), they will expect to fail these tasks in the future. Failing at a task one thinks one should be able to control is the leading cause for feelings of humiliation, shame, and anger. Shame comes from devaluing oneself, which often exacerbates poor performance. Feelings of hopelessness result.

On the other hand, a method reinforcing an internal locus of control enhances feelings of success while diminishing feelings of failure. Greater feelings of self-efficacy contribute to and enhance one's self-esteem.

In the past, Deidre had the habit of controlling stress by eating chocolate, which always concomitantly provoked a negative self-image. Eating chocolate meant she was out of control and doing something bad. Based on attribution theory, her self-perception was that eating chocolate meant she was a bad person. Whenever she was stressed out, she ate chocolate, which heightened her feelings of being out of control—the root of most of her self-disrespect.

Deidre was now learning strategies to develop a stronger cause-and-effect relationship that linked her newly emerging self-efficacy and her performance outcomes. In spite of difficult situations, she continued working toward her goals. She did not eat her contract food. Voluntarily giving up chocolate created an internal locus of control over this previously uncontrollable food. Adhering to her contract enabled Deidre to begin learning how to engage and rely on what's defined as an intrinsic motivator. Those relying on intrinsic-type thinking have greater feelings of self-control, and self-control promotes self-confidence.

Not eating one specific highly enjoyable food that she had always turned to for self-soothing allowed Deidre to observe and therefore change underlying cognitive dimensions about current eating patterns while being confident about being able to resolve whatever problem might arise in her future. Skills were being set in place that enabled her to devise solution-oriented strategies in spite of occasional missed expectations.

SALIVARY EXTINCTION ELIMINATES NONCOMPLIANCE

At this point, Deidre hasn't eaten chocolate for more than three months. Applying Pavlov's extinction curve for this elapsed time, a person will be desensitized to whatever item was given up, hence the incoming data (i.e., the contract food) will fail to evoke a reaction (bodily/emotional response). In scientific terms, Deidre now benefits from what's called a *convincing indicator*—control over one particular behavior has been accomplished. If the right contract food is given up, observing and changing other cognitive dimensions for a variety of eating patterns becomes feasible.

After three months, Deidre was confident she was capable of keeping self-monitoring skills at the ready at all times. Whatever might happen in every other area of her life, not eating chocolate helped her continue to experience a sense of control—a paradise of the mind, if you will—always at her disposal. For Deidre, not eating chocolate fostered the positive modification of behaviors in all areas of her life.

In the following chapter, you will find out whether the physiological extinction of Deidre's craving for chocolate subsequently gave her the ability to meet and manage the emotional war she faced on her next birthday.

17

$\blacklozenge$

THE PINK BOX REVISITED

It was November 13th, Deidre's birthday, and almost six months to the day since she hadn't eaten her contract food. In pre-ICP days, Deidre's craving for chocolate would have prevailed and made the decision to eat her birthday cake a done deal. But now, her cravings for chocolate had been extinguished. Even though her contract specifically provided an exemption for her birthday, the thought of eating a chocolate birthday cake filled her with trepidation about eating a previously out-of-control food item.

Deidre arrived at her mom's house, unlocked the front door, and yelled, "Hi Mom, I'm here." Her mother's expected response came drifting down from upstairs. "The birthday girl is here! Don't look inside the Pink Box. I don't want my surprise spoiled!"

Slowly, Deidre walked through the living room toward the kitchen. On the counter sat the Pink Box. Knowing what the box contained, she opened it nonetheless and came face-to-face with the iconic seven-layer chocolate cake, a sight that would previously have led to an inevitable downfall if Deidre were on any other weight-loss program.

MODIFICATION OF ONE EATING BEHAVIOR

How did Deidre's contract food relate to her embedded feelings associated with dieting? The birthday cake had assumed symbolic proportions; its annual presence served as a focal point in her personal battle of the bulge and provided Deidre with an opportunity to assess the role that salivary extinction (i.e., the extinction of the craving response) would play in deciding whether to temporarily reintroduce or not reintroduce chocolate back into her life.

Each day that passed since making her contract, Deidre had become more and more confident that having not eaten chocolate made adherence to the ICP easier. In her own words, "It feels like I breezed through my three-month mark, realizing it was effortless since I wasn't fighting chocolate cravings. Yes, I did have a brief episode when I felt bad, but I got through it. Now, it doesn't seem as if I'm in a constant food battle. I'm also not feeling guilty and ashamed about my food choices anymore."

Craving responses destabilize the process of making conscious, astute decisions about your food options. As far as Deidre was concerned, continually fighting chocolate cravings had made her feel as if her body were her enemy. But having not eaten chocolate for six months convinced her that she had choices. Deidre now viewed her commitment to maintaining her contract food obligation as an ally, a supportive friend who would help her in times of need. Again, upholding her contract was the reason she had been able to exceed the three-month mark, a point that had always bedeviled her when pursuing every other weight-loss program. This realization greatly enhanced Deidre's confidence in herself and in the ICP. And she realized that she had chosen wisely about what food item to give up. It was irrefutable that she had always turned to chocolate at some point in every other dieting protocol, which had sealed her fate and had invariably triggered an unrecoverable relapse.

As her birthday approached, Deidre began experiencing a great deal of anxiety about the cake. The closer her birthday came, the more uncomfortable she felt about the thought of temporarily reintroducing her contract food into her life. She began to worry that once she began eating it again she'd never be able forestall an unrecoverable relapse, as had always happened in the past.

Adapting to the pressure of following food rules combined with the pressures of meeting her mom's needs and expectations had previously convinced Deidre there was no such thing as free will when the time came to go on a diet. These kinds of mind games are just not possible with the ICP. Eating chocolate cake on her birthday had been her intention right from the start of her involvement in the program—a decision she made willingly and voluntarily. This would make it impossible for her to blame her mom or anyone else if she ate the cake and experienced an unrecoverable relapse, since the decision about whether to partake of the contents of the Pink Box would be hers and hers alone. On her birthday, Deidre would be in the position of taking complete responsibility for eating or not eating chocolate cake.

Deidre's feelings of anticipatory trepidation about this decision-making moment escalated in late October. She knew she would soon have to decide whether to eat her chocolate birthday cake. For the last few months, she'd been expressing that she had no desire to eat chocolate. If it were served, it would be effortless for her to turn it down. Deidre began saying that if she was eating out with friends, she actually hoped they'd order something chocolate for dessert so she could have practice declining, and it would also make her feel good about "banking" the dessert calories for future meals.

The dilemma Deidre now faced was that she knew how devastated her mom would be if she didn't partake in the entire birthday experience, one that had become a choreographed family tradition. Eating the birthday cake would surely meet her mom's needs and expectations, but Deidre still couldn't allay her fears that there was a good chance it would reignite a craving response for chocolate and trigger an unrecoverable relapse.

Deidre was beginning to see the bigger problem. Having firsthand knowledge, her experience told her that by not eating one immensely enjoyable food, she was successfully managing other high-risk behaviors. The link was clear. Something that had always been unattainable (i.e., resisting binge eating by exclusively resorting to willpower) was now attainable by the simple act of giving up one problematic food—chocolate. Not having to enlist willpower for her contract food also encouraged greater introspection about her eating patterns.

Yes, the deviation for the chocolate birthday cake had been specifically built into Deidre's contract from the get-go, and she had prepared herself for this temporary indulgence. But I also concurred that it could lead to an irreversible regression, because it only took one paired-association to restimulate a full-force craving response. This would make it less likely that Deidre could continue to rely on her newly found skills to counteract any potential relapse. Ultimately, it was Deidre's choice and her choice alone.

THE CONTRACT FOOD ITEM PRODUCES SELF-DIRECTEDNESS

If the correct food is chosen from the outset, the ICP experience of deconditioning the craving response promotes the kind of self-reflection required to make positive behavioral changes regarding current and future eating patterns. Specifically, the extinction of one craving response becomes the measurable enhancer of self-evaluations skills. For Deidre, not craving chocolate provided a whole new experience in the way she spoke to herself about herself. The ultimate goal is to initiate a sort of self-directed introspective monologue that objectively weighs the pros and cons in order to make better food choices. When Deidre made food decisions now, she could simply compare her self-control established by not eating the contract food with her previous out-of-control eating patterns.

Deidre began to realize that while food in the mouth works to self-soothe, the effects are short-lived. Many other eating patterns were becoming discernible, because she no longer had to continually fight her chocolate cravings. This is what convinced her that if the ICP didn't work for her, nothing would; she felt this was her last chance for weight-loss success. It was evident that Deidre had chosen the correct food to give up; during the last six months, any time she felt that she had gone off track, she had quickly recovered. All long-term damage was averted, and every regression was easily managed because of the sense of accomplishment engendered by having not eaten her contract food.

DID DEIDRE'S EMOTIONAL RESPONSE TO CHOCOLATE PREVAIL?

In all her previous dieting attempts, Deidre had been able to justify eating something considered off her diet by rationalizing that she wasn't really responsible because someone else was to blame (e.g., her mother). The external pressure from her mom was Deidre's justification for deluding herself into feeling incapable of taking responsibility for eating the contents of the Pink Box. Bottom line: the decision to partake from the Pink Box was a voluntary act that, in reality, made it patently unreasonable for Deidre to blame her mom or anyone else for her decision. For Deidre, this propensity to rationalize and deny responsibility was no longer an issue; the ICP has been strategically designed so that it's impossible to argue that outside pressures are to blame for one's own decision-making missteps.

It was now Deidre's birthday, and the time had finally come for her to make her Pink Box decision. As she stared at the seven-layer chocolate cake, she reflected on the control she had established by not eating her contract food and compared her current behaviors with the out-of-control eating patterns that chocolate had previously evoked. She realized that responsibility for her food behaviors was hers alone. Deidre made her decision. She reached into the Pink Box and gently took out the birthday cake. Then she walked over to the sink, turned on the water, and shoved the cake down the garbage disposal—irrefutable proof that she had achieved quintessential self-directedness.

EPILOGUE

As discussed throughout this book, if people ate when hungry and stopped when sated, they'd have no weight problem. For most of us, however, the immediate gratification of food consumption is an undeniable factor that, from a physical and/or emotional perspective, motivates overeating episodes. People very often eat to self-soothe even when they are not hungry, which is antithetical to the dictates handed down by so-called experts in the dieting industry.

Another example of the difference between the ICP methodology and the dictates imposed by traditional diet and weight-loss programs relates to eating schedules. The dieting industry insists that dieters adopt eating schedules incorporating the following rules, which are presumably derived from the results of legitimate experimentation. First and foremost, breakfast is considered imperative. Dieters who snack between meals with anything other than fruits or vegetables have no chance of success. Nighttime eating is considered taboo. Skipping meals is a no-no, because you'll get too hungry. Such rules develop into an internalized stimulus-response mechanism that underscores how noncompliant acts trigger anxiety. Failing to incorporate these rules into one's eating schedule often leads to negative feelings resulting from having broken the rules, which creates a vicious circle of noncompliance that the overweight person is unable to escape. In contrast, the ICP encourages you to research eating schedules in order to determine what works best for you.

The ICP incorporates the dynamics of two scientific learning principles—classical conditioning and operant conditioning—into a methodology that enables you to decrease the frequency and caloric magnitude of nonhunger-eating events. Utilizing the single-subject research design, this methodology helps you transition from the traditional dieting mentality of relying on an external locus of control (which is ineffective over the long term) to an internal locus of control (which is necessary to achieve lifelong weight management). Utilizing both principles will provide the advantage of being able to think more rationally and conscientiously about your food choices. A review of how these two principles work in tandem follows.

THE FOOD CONTRACT USES THE PRINCIPLE OF CLASSICAL CONDITIONING

The ICP incorporates the dynamics of classical conditioning by means of a contract to give up one problematic food.

The sight or smell of food (even after eating a large meal) is categorized as an external stimulus. The hyper responsiveness to a highly palatable item often triggers brain function that causes a wide variety of bodily reactions, such as pupil dilation and salivary response (to name only two). Such reactions are classically conditioned responses—specialized responses within the body from smooth muscle activity. Dieting experts have always considered these smooth-muscle reactions to incoming food data to be automatic/ reflexive and, therefore, not within one's control.

A highly enjoyable food that typically evokes an automatic/reflexive smooth-muscle reaction doesn't necessarily mean you will eat the food. You smell and/or see a yummy food, and you want it. But responding to external stimuli by actually eating the food can't happen without striated or operant conditioning types of muscle activity. Getting up to get the food, wrapping your fingers around a serving spoon, using a fork to put the food in your mouth, chewing, keeping your lips closed so food doesn't fall out of your mouth, moving your tongue, and swallowing food involve striated rather than smooth muscles. Striated muscles are within your control.

In its most fundamental aspect, the contract to give up one problematic food uses the principle of classical conditioning. The food contract is based on clinical application of Pavlov's research, which shows that classically conditioned craving responses to a particular food (e.g., salivation) can be extinguished by giving up that item.

Secondarily, giving up one problematic food not only helps you transform decision-making from an external to an internal locus of control but also ultimately helps you distinguish between feelings of hunger and appetite. You begin to increase the frequency of eating in response to hunger while decreasing the frequency of eating in response to environmental cues. Extinction of a craving response allows you to assess with greater sensitivity the internal physiological cues that comprise the basis for an empirical evaluation of the bodily sensations that have historically prompted your overeating behaviors.

THE FOOD LEDGER USES THE PRINCIPLE OF OPERANT CONDITIONING

The ICP incorporates the dynamics of operant conditioning by means of a food-consumption ledger.

At its most fundamental level, the ledger uses the principle of operant conditioning. Writing down details in the ledger before eating is an operant that eliminates the possibility of automatic and/or nonthinking food choices. Picking up a pen and writing down what you intend to eat requires the use of striated muscles—actions that are within your control. Writing down what you are about to eat before you eat it employs the ultimate operant conditioning technique for attaining behavioral changes.

Secondarily, the ledger helps you to take responsibility for all your eating behaviors and provides the information necessary to research solutions to counterproductive food decisions and eating situations. Feelings, thoughts, and behaviors become more visible through this method of personalized investigative inquiry, which leads to minimizing the frequency and caloric magnitude of overeating episodes. Fewer lapses (i.e., weight-gain days) are likely to occur, and when they do, they can form the basis for new learning. Using the ledger also facilitates a cognitive distinction between hunger and appetite. Rating hunger and preference often helps you realize that you're not really hungry. This leads to increased feelings of control, allowing you to gradually increase responsibility by learning to more accurately assess bodily sensations. Ledger keeping encourages the evaluation of progress toward your weight-loss goal by making personal data visible. It provides the means for you to access food-related experiences in order to learn more about yourself and the way you eat. You are taking an action within your control when you use the ledger.

CONTROLLING HUNGER IS NOT THE SOLUTION FOR PERMANENT WEIGHT MANAGEMENT

The ICP embodies the reality that most overeating episodes resulting in weight gain are the result of eating to self-soothe rather than to satiate hunger. Eating habits are learned and persist as the result of repeated correlations made from thoughts and emotions associated with pleasurable foods. Food associations become embedded into everyone's modus operandi, as do craving responses for self-soothing purposes. In order to manage your relationship with food, one fact must be acknowledged: eating as a way to cope with discomfort works!

Research reveals that sucking and chewing are instinctively soothing. Evidence in the womb shows the sucking reflex occurs as early as thirty-two weeks into gestation. A reflex results from an inborn impulse initiating in the nerve centers of the brain. Sucking behavior is an automatic (i.e., nonthinking) reaction; it is an instinctual self-soothing behavior. As we continue to develop, sucking for self-soothing extends to chewing for self-soothing. The mere act of chewing food feels good. Sucking and chewing actions become associated with a stimulus (e.g., any stressor) and serve as a coping mechanism. In effect, they serve as the equivalent of adult pacifiers. As we continue to mature, specific and highly desirable foods become factored into the comfort equation. This sucking and chewing action for comfort most often has nothing whatsoever to do with physiological hunger.

Problematic eating patterns are formed based on the effect that certain foods have on different emotional states. When we eat certain enjoyable foods in response to familiar emotional states, we develop a craving for those foods as a coping strategy. Highly preferable foods are chosen for a reason—we choose foods that will give us the greatest bang for the buck. Specific foods then become correlated with specific emotional states, resulting in food cravings that evolve into highly individualized habits. That is, highly preferable foods eaten over and over again are the basis for all our problematic eating patterns. These eating habits put us at a disadvantage for staying on track with our weight-loss and -management goals. Following this precept, you'll begin to appreciate the small role hunger plays when it comes to weight reduction and weight-loss sustainability.

Based upon the notion that controlling hunger is the cure for long-term weight reduction, most weight-loss programs attempt to manage overeating and deter people from using food for comfort by providing rigid guidelines about what are and are not acceptable food choices. Because dieters believe that eating when not hungry is taboo, eating as a means to self-soothe most often leads to the downfall of any dieting attempt. The moment a dieter eats to self-soothe, he or she has gone off the diet. The diet is over, and an unrecoverable relapse sets in.

The fact is that controlling hunger doesn't have much to do with weight reduction and weight-loss sustainability. It is true that allowing oneself to get too hungry can be problematic, because it can cause overconsumption. However, not getting too hungry is simple to manage, because hunger naturally drives us to eat. Again, what is most often problematic about our food choices is using food as a coping mechanism and not to satiate hunger. Food in the mouth feels good, it's convenient, and it's one of the most common—if not the most efficient—ways to cope with stressors. Yet if controlling hunger isn't the solution for weight loss or weight-loss maintenance, what is?

THE ICP METHODOLOGY IS THE SOLUTION FOR PERMANENT WEIGHT MANAGEMENT

The answer for permanent weight management combines the classical conditioning principle of salivary extinction for a single out-of-control food item with a proven operant-conditioning methodology incorporating the reality that eating is a natural way to self-soothe. Because food habits and cravings are learned, they can be unlearned through application of these two scientifically based learning principles. The ICP methodology strategically uses both principles in tandem to help you reach your weight-loss goal and provides the foundation for lifelong weight management.

I often refer to a concept I call the "assassination of craving responses." Foods that were once problematic can now be easily managed by determining the frequency with which they are eaten based on ledger keeping. Some clients find that, over the years, they may need to add other items to their food contract.

It is clear that for successful weight loss and weight-loss maintenance to occur, one must manage eating behaviors that are typically dictated not so much by hunger as by environmental cues. Do I want to eat three meals a day? If I'm not hungry, should I eat? Does snacking lead to overeating? What food schedule should I follow for me to lose weight successfully?

Everything written so far implies two simple equations—if hungry, eat; if not hungry, it's okay to not eat. If you're not hungry but you want to eat, make decisions that won't end up making you feel bad. If you do feel bad about a decision, you'll at least know that you haven't eaten your contract food and that you've written in your ledger. In this way, positive feelings will be maintained, and in the process, you'll also be decreasing the frequency and magnitude of high-calorie days. You design an eating schedule based on your particular needs by focusing on specific problems and experiences in order to control your particular problematic eating behaviors. Be your own guide, and follow a schedule that works best for you.

Adherence to both requirements of the ICP enables weight management through the identification of problematic foods and the development of potential solutions to problematic eating situations. Although feelings about eating patterns can change quite quickly, behavioral changes require practice before they become habits. Using the food contract and the food-consumption ledger in tandem helps you to learn to assess more accurately what hunger actually is and to objectively evaluate how you make your food choices. Confidence in the ability to control your eating behaviors facilitates attainment of the ultimate goal of this program—to minimize the caloric magnitude and frequency of regressions.

By incorporating a proven methodology based on scientific learning principles, the ICP takes off where every other weight-loss method falls short—namely, the handling of a regression. Permanent weight management requires major attitude and lifestyle changes. Each person must develop fundamental attitude changes, learn more positive coping skills, and maximize a sense of personal control. When a regression does happen, how it's dealt with determines whether or not the lapse will become permanent. In contrast to other programs that do not address this critically important issue, the scientific method of investigation—at the very core of the ICP methodology—has repeatedly and unequivocally demonstrated its efficacy in managing the all-but-inevitable regressions that are part and parcel of losing weight.

Compared to willpower, the effortlessness of avoiding eating the contract food and recording data in the ledger are what will furnish you with an uplifting sense of confidence and competence when it comes to your self-management skills. Ideally, accurate attention to how your body is responding to your food choices and food experiences will also generate more effective decision-making strategies in other areas of your life, enabling you (like Deidre) to achieve quintessential self-directedness, a laudable goal in a life replete with choices and an array of tempting Pink Boxes.

POSTSCRIPT:
A CLIENT'S VIEW OF THE LEDGER

For those who are committed
To regaining their self-control
Over negative eating habits
That have taken a serious toll.

The Ledger is a research tool
With the very real potential
To enable self-awareness
Leading to changes that are essential.

Its method is straightforward
But requires nothing less
Than the highest degree of compliance
To achieve what it promises.

Each time, before you eat your food
You create a frame of reference
By writing the date, the time, the place
The calories, hunger, and preference.

From this exercise, you will derive
Much valuable information
And insight to effect in yourself
A positive transformation.

Technicality is critical
For therein lies the key
To extracting the fullest feedback
From each and every entry.

But never forget to forgive yourself
For occasional slips you may make
None of us is perfect
And we can learn from each mistake.

You'll receive ongoing reinforcement
As you see your efforts lead
Toward continual growth and progress
And the knowledge you can succeed.

Ultimately, for the work you've done
The Ledger will reward you
With attainment of the goals you've set
And a healthier life to look forward to.

MEET DEENA SOLOMON, PHD, MFT

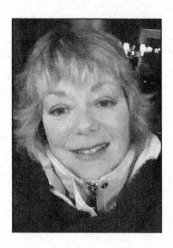

She received her M.S. in Counseling Psychology in 1983 from California State University Los Angeles in 1983 and was awarded a Doctorate in Psychology in 1991 from the California Graduate Institute (now named the Chicago School of Professional Psychology in Los Angeles). She subsequently continued her post-doctoral studies for three years and earned her Behavioral Medicine Certification in 1994. A licensed clinical psychotherapist, she served on the California Board of Behavioral Science Examiners and was assigned the title of expert examiner. Dr. Solomon has worked as a clinician in the field of weight loss and weight loss management for more than three decades and has developed a proprietary scientifically based and scientifically proven methodology for helping disheartened dieters attain and maintain their weight reduction goals.

CPSIA information can be obtained
at www.ICGtesting.com
Printed in the USA
BVOW09s1930160617

487083BV00001B/1/P